MW01230726

Intermittent Fasting 16/8

Cookbook with Easy to Follow and Delicious Recipes.

Includes:

Meal Plan For 2 Weeks to Prepare You For Your Journey

Calorie Count On Each Recipe

by VL DeAlexander

Copyright © 2019 VL DeAlexander

All rights reserved.

Please note that the information contained within this document is for educational and entertainment purposes only. All effort has been executed to present accurate, up to date, and reliable, complete information. No warranties of any kind are declared or implied. Readers acknowledge that the author is not engaging in the rendering of legal, financial, medical or professional advice. The content within this book has been derived from various sources. Please consult a licensed professional before attempting any techniques outlined in this book.

ISBN-13: 978-1-0747-5912-4

CONTENTS

1 Introduction   1

2 A Quick Overview Of The 16:8   4
Intermittent Fasting Method

3 The Benefits Of 16:8 Intermittent Fasting   7
For Your Health

4 How Intermittent Fasting Is Used For   11
Weight Loss

How Weight Loss Is Achieved In General?

Intermittent Fasting And Weight Loss Through a
Caloric Deficit

5 Setting-Up Your Two-Week Intermittent   16
Fasting Meal Plan

Understand Your Goals And Know What You Are
Aiming For

Decide When To Eat And When To Fast

Calculate Your Ideal Daily Caloric Intake

6 Calorie Goal Formula   27

Determine What Foods You Should Include In
Your Meal Plan

7   Intermittent Fasting Meals   34

8   Two-Week Intermittent Fasting Meal Plan   37

9   Weight Loss Recipes For Your Intermittent   46
    Fasting Program

10 Extra Tips To Get The Most Out Of   73
    Intermittent Fasting

    Adjust Your Diet Plan As You Go

    Don't Overlook The Importance Of Exercise In a
    Weight Loss Strategy

    Deal With Hunger Pang Like a Boss

    Avoid Eating These Foods

11 Conclusion   81

CHAPTER 1

INTRODUCTION

More than half of the entire world's population is overweight. Think about that for just a second – it is alarming how quickly the prevalence of obesity and overweight has grown in just the last 30 years or so. This increasing trend of obesity and people who are overweight has also led to the dieting and supplement industry exploiting this as an opportunity for them to gain billions in profit – often promoting products that are worthless and ineffective when it comes to losing excess fat that has been stored in the body.

Even though there are so many weight loss programs and pills on the market that is not supported by scientific studies or evidence, and often yields results that are not desirable, all is not lost.

There are strategies that have been proven

effective for long-term weight loss. When you follow a well-planned strategy, you will be able to lose weight safely (losing weight too quickly is harmful) – and you will be able to keep that weight off for the years to come, as long as you assure you implement appropriate healthy lifestyle habits and continue to follow them.

One particular strategy that has become popular among people who are trying to live a healthier life and lose weight at the same time is intermittent fasting.

Intermittent fasting is a technique that relies on fasting for a period of time and then having a relatively small eating window, where all meals of the day should be fitted into.

Even though scientific studies have yielded evidence that has proven intermittent fasting to be an effective weight loss tool, it should also be noted that not planning an appropriate strategy and implementing a meal plan that focuses on weight loss will not yield the results that you might be aiming for.

The reason you have picked up this book is probably that you have tried multiple diets and found that the success rate is often not something to be desired. It's true – most of the diets out there fail. Many of these diets do not only fail but causes complications once you stop following the program. For many people, extra weight gain is a very unpleasant complication that they suffer after they have undergone a diet program.

You have probably heard about intermittent fasting and that it has yielded positive results for thousands of people in the past. Scientific data has already proven this. Yet, you are not sure how to get started, where to start, when to eat, which program to follow, and, of course, what to eat.

If this is you, don't fret. In this book, you'll discover a complete guide to what you should eat, how you need to calculate a desirable caloric intake, how much you should eat, and I'll share with you some of the most important reasons why the intermittent fasting diet plays such a crucial role in getting your body on track and to lose weight in a healthy way.

For those who do not know much about intermittent fasting, apart from the fact that it has helped a lot of people lose weight, I'll start this book by providing a quick overview of intermittent fasting in general, as well as the specific intermittent fasting method that we will be focusing on in this guide. I'll also give you a brief overview of how to determine what you should eat for the goal that you have in mind, and give you an overview of various options that you can choose from when it comes to preparing meals (that are delicious, by the way).

CHAPTER 2

A QUICK OVERVIEW OF THE 16:8 INTERMITTENT FASTING METHOD

Let's start this book by taking just a quick look at intermittent fasting and the 16:8 method. There are many options that you can opt for if you wish to follow an intermittent fasting plan, but for most people, the 16:8 method is the best option. This particular method is especially useful for beginners who will be fasting for the very first time. It holds fewer risks, and you will spend less time trying to figure out when is the best time to eat and what exactly you should eat.

Intermittent fasting, in general, is a technique used where you get a relatively small window during the day when you are allowed to eat. For the rest of the day, you will fast. What this means is that you will basically only rely on water while fasting.

A variety of intermittent fasting techniques have been developed, with some of them being quite complex and requires a lot of initial planning to avoid malnutrition or other potential complications.

We will be focusing on the 16:8 method in this book, as I have previously mentioned. The reason for this is simple. The 16:8 method was designed to provide a good overview and feeling of what intermittent fasting holds and gives you a solid plan to work with. This is the most uncomplicated option that you can opt for, and it will not cause you to feel excessive hunger or like you are starving yourself.

The 16:8 intermittent fasting the day into two sections – this includes the fasting window and the eating window. It is quite similar to many of the other methods that have been developed but offers a better balance in terms of these two windows.

The method includes an eight-hour eating window, along with a 16-hour fasting window in each 24-hour cycle.

This means that if you are used to eating three meals each day, for example, you will have to squeeze those three meals into the eight-hour eating window that you get, as you are allowed water primarily during the period that you need to fast.

Sure, not being allowed to eat for 16 hours of the day might sound a little harsh. Many people who do research on this method of intermittent fasting think that they will be starving themselves and will always feel hungry. It's normal to think this if you have never actually tried fasting yourself.

If you are wondering if you will feel hungry all the time, then the answer to the question is really both yes and no. At first, it might take some self-control and patience in order to get used to this new way of eating and to let your body adjust to the new schedule that you are following.

Once you get used to the 16:8 intermittent fasting method, however, you will find that those hunger pangs that come on so early in the morning start to disappear. Cravings won't be as much of a problem anymore – which is certainly a huge benefit for people who often find themselves craving for something sweet in the afternoon.

CHAPTER 3

THE BENEFITS OF 16:8 INTERMITTENT FASTING FOR YOUR HEALTH

Intermittent fasting techniques, including the 16:8 method, are most commonly used to assist in weight loss by the general population. The method has been tried by thousands of people and also scientifically proven to be a helpful resource in reducing body fat and improving body composition. Weight loss is often considered the number one reason why people opt for a diet and program that utilizes intermittent fasting, in fact.

While a reduction in body fat is definitely one of the best advantages to be mentioned in terms of intermittent fasting, there are more advantages that people gain when they decide that they are going to follow this type of program – especially if they truly commit to it and can implement self-control that ensures they do not give in to cravings.

Intermittent fasting is known to assist in improving your body composition as well, as I mentioned earlier. Body composition refers to a series of features – this includes your body fat percentage and lean muscle mass primarily. A program that utilizes intermittent fasting, along with an appropriate diet plan, will bring down your body fat percentage, and push up your lean muscle mass at the same time.

It is also important to note the benefits that are associated with weight loss for people with an excessive amount of fat distributed throughout their body. Since overweight and obesity is linked to so many chronic diseases that can truly make your life dreadful, losing even small amounts of weight can drastically reduce your risk of these diseases. Additionally, if you have already been diagnosed with a disease associated with obesity, reduced body weight may improve the symptoms that you are experiencing and help you get the disease under control.

Take type 2 diabetes, for example. In one study, scientists describe that factors such as proinflammatory markers, cytokines, hormones, glycerol, and non-esterified fatty acids are all increased among those people who are obese. In turn, these factors all have factors that link them to insulin resistance. When insulin resistance develops, it can continue to progress into type 2 diabetes if the affected person does not implement appropriate preventative measures.

When you develop type 2 diabetes, you become predisposed to many additional risks and complications. In fact, type 2 diabetes can cause severe complications that may not only lead to disability but also become life-threatening. This disease can also affect all of the body's most important organs, including the heart, and can damage various tissues, such as nerves, throughout the body.

In addition to assisting in reducing body weight and bringing down the risks associated with obesity, intermittent fasting has many other benefits that are also worth mentioning.

Through intermittent fasting, cellular changes may occur in the body. This can lead to levels of human growth hormones rising by as much as 500%. This leads to a faster rate of fat burning, while also producing an increase in muscle mass.

It has also been found that intermittent fasting can help to remove waste that has built up in cells within the human body and can also assist in the repair process of cells that have been damaged. This means cells in the body become more efficient in performing their specialized functions.

One study also explains how recent findings from scientists suggest that intermittent fasting helps to improve brain health and may play a crucial role in helping medical experts better understand how diseases like Parkinson's disease and Alzheimer's disease can be prevented in the future.

Furthermore, following an intermittent fasting plan can also help to reduce levels of inflammation within the human body, as well as help to fight against oxidative stress. Both of these factors are known to contribute to numerous chronic diseases significantly and can causes certain molecules to become damaged, which can inhibit their functionality within the body.

In one study, scientists tested how intermittent fasting would work on the brain health and cardiovascular health among a group of laboratory rats. They found significant improvements in various tests used to determine the well-being of these two crucial hormones of the body. The scientists also associated these improvements among the tested laboratory rats with the reduction in oxidative stress that were observed. Additionally, the scientists also observed an improvement in the cellular stress resistance ratings in these rats. What this means is that an intermittent fasting diet can help to reduce the effect that stress has on the body, and help to fight against the existing oxidative damage, often also referred to as free radical damage, that has already occurred.

CHAPTER 4

HOW INTERMITTENT FASTING IS USED FOR WEIGHT LOSS

You understand the benefits that 16:8 intermittent fasting has in store for you, so now you might be asking how exactly is this type of fasting program used for the purpose of losing weight. I have both good news and bad news to share with you here.

The process of using intermittent fasting to help you shed excess fat is actually quite simple, but only if you have the right tools and guidance at your disposal. You cannot just decide to start fasting for the first part of the day and continue to eat as many donuts as you can possibly stuff into your mouth when you reach your eating window. This is a recipe for disaster. You'll end up gaining weight instead of losing weight!

In this section, I'll tell you more about how intermittent fasting should be used, along with both diet and an appropriate program to ensure you can burn calories, for weight loss. I'll break the entire process down into multiple steps so that you can better understand where to start and how the entire program should work in order to yield the results that you desire.

How Weight Loss Is Achieved in General?

Before we look at the best way that you can use intermittent fasting to help you reduce your body fat percentage, let's first quickly consider how weight loss generally works – think of this as the science behind effective and guaranteed weight loss.

When you eat something – regardless of what it is – it means you are putting calories into your body. Nutrients are broken down and absorbed by your body, while carbohydrates are broken down and then processed into glucose, which is then distributed through your body to provide cells with energy.

When excess glucose is present in your body, it will usually be stored as fat cells through a rather complicated process that we are not going to be discussing in detail here. As fat cells increase, you gain weight – ultimately leading to you becoming overweight and then slowly obese.

Now, on the other hand, when you are physically active – whether you are walking, dancing, or going hard on the treadmill at the gym – you are burning calories. Your body uses more glucose for energy, and when the reserves run out, the body starts looking toward stored fat cells in order to generate more energy. This energy then allows you to continue running on that treadmill or allows you to pick up the set of weights a few more times.

So, to sum this up – you eat, you gain calories; you exercise, you lose calories.

When the number of calories you eat surpasses the number of calories you lose, then you gain weight. Think of this within a 24-hour cycle. If you eat 2,000 calories, but only burn 1,000, then you gain weight to the value of those extra 1,000 calories that are left behind at the end of the day.

When you eat more calories than you burn, it means there is a caloric surplus. You are gaining weight and cannot lose weight with this strategy.

To lose weight, this entire equation needs to be in an opposite manner. You need to lose more calories than you burn. If you eat food that calculates to around 2,000 calories each day, you need to burn more than the 2,000 calories if you wish ever to see your fat go away and the number of the scale go down.

When your daily calorie intake is less than the number of calories you lose, then it means you have a caloric deficit – this is the ideal goal that you are striving toward when you are aiming to reduce your body weight.

Intermittent Fasting and Weight Loss Through a Caloric Deficit

You should have a basic understanding of how weight loss works – that you need to create a caloric deficit if you ever wish to see your weight go down.

Now, let's take a quick look at how intermittent fasting plays a role in this entire process. With intermittent fasting, you still need to create a caloric deficit. I've seen some people think that simply because they are fasting, they will lose weight, regardless of the other factors in their life. This is not true.

No matter how beneficial fasting might be and a program that utilizes intermittent fasting, you will still need to take the science behind weight loss into account. If your caloric intake is more than how many calories you lose in a day, then you set the way for weight gain and not weight loss.

Intermittent fasting can make things a little easier, however. It has been found that people who follow an intermittent fasting program eventually experience improvements in their level of satiety. Their appetite is reduced, in other words. Since weight gain often lies within the fact that a person is unable to control their urges to eat inappropriate times, the reduced appetite will certainly be beneficial.

Additionally, because all meals of the day need to be squeezed into an eight-hour window with the particular intermittent fasting method that I am focusing on in this guide, it usually means that you will still feel somewhat full with your second meal after you had your first. When the time comes to have your third meal, the second meal will still be satisfying your appetite a little. You'll end up not wanting to overload your plate every chance you get – this means it becomes much, much easier than before to be in control of how many calories you will be consuming on a day-to-day basis.

Now, combine this with exercise. You won't even have to hit the gym too hard and may even be able to burn an adequate number of calories exercising at home if you are able to reduce the number of calories you consume by simply feeling full from the last meal when the time for the next meal comes.

CHAPTER 5

SETTING UP YOUR TWO-WEEK INTERMITTENT FASTING MEAL PLAN

Now we're at the part where we start to take action. I've told you about why intermittent fasting is a great option that you should consider, how this plan will help you, and how intermittent fasting should ideally be used in order to help you achieve successful weight loss results.

We are now moving on to the process of setting up a meal plan for the next two weeks. Even though we are only focusing on two weeks in this book, this will give you a good taste of what intermittent fasting holds, how the program can benefit you, what you can do with such a program, and it will help you decide if this is an appropriate type of eating plan that you would want to follow.

Once you have completed the initial two-week

period of intermittent fasting, you can decide if you want to go ahead and extend your program. At this time, you can continue with the plan that you have developed for yourself (I will provide you with a great program in this book, so don't worry if you're not sure how to develop your own meal plan), or rather make some adjustments in order to better accompany your specific body and, of course, your goals.

Getting started is really the hardest part – and I believe that initial planning can really make things much easier. When you are organized and know what to eat and when to eat, you won't have to find yourself in chaos, unsure of what you will be preparing for dinner or any other meal. You will be able to have a stress-free two weeks, knowing exactly how your day will go – at least in terms of food, that is.

I am going to go through the process of setting up your intermittent fasting meal plan below. I will also provide you with some excellent recipes that you can follow in the next section – you will have to combine these two sections in order to determine what meals you should eat and when you should eat these meals. There is a lot of personal choices that will be implemented here, so the way you will be implementing an intermittent fasting program in your own life can likely defer from the next person's plans.

Understand Your Goals and Know What You Are Aiming For

We'll start off by taking a look at the goals that you are trying to achieve, what you are aiming for with the intermittent fasting diet that you are looking to start implementing in your life. Okay, I know – you picked up this book because you saw that it is about using intermittent fasting for weight loss. You were not wrong, but the thing is, every person has different goals even when it comes to a specific topic like losing weight.

For example, a person who is obese will have to adopt a stricter diet and often include a larger caloric deficit, as well as understand that they will need to follow their diet plan for a more significant period of time, compared to someone who is only overweight and needs to lose just a few pounds.

Start by getting on the scale. Take down your current weight and consider your height – use a BMI calculator to help you determine if you are overweight, obese, or perhaps even morbidly obese.

Do not only look at your weight. Consider your personal goals as well. Are you trying to lose weight over a period of time in order to gradually adopt a healthier lifestyle and avoid the dreadful diseases that are associated with excess weight in the body? Or do you have an upcoming event that you would like to lose some weight for, as you really want to fit into a specific dress or a pair of jeans, but need to come down a size or two to do so?

As you can see, things can quickly become complicated here. Write down your weight, your BMI, and your goals.

Another question to ask yourself is whether you would like to build lean muscle mass within your fat burning program, or rather only focus on losing your excess weight for the time being, and then, later on, implement a program to assist with your body composition.

When you wish to build some muscle while following this program, you will likely need to make a few alterations to a standard diet. In addition to a caloric deficit, you'll have to include specific types of nutrients in your diet, which can often be obtained with the use of supplements, in order to accelerate muscle growth – you will, of course, also need to participate in appropriate strength training exercises.

In this book, I am primarily focusing on weight loss, but I will include a few tips that you can use, such as recommendations on specific supplements, if you have additional goals that you would like to include in your diet. I'll also tell you how you can calculate exactly how many calories and what types of foods you should eat in order to ensure you are able to get the best chance possible of reaching your goals in a minimal time period.

Decide When to Eat and When to Fast

You now know your goals and have them written down, hopefully in the same file that you will be using to set up your intermittent fasting meal plan and track your progress. Before you continue with the process and start actually to set up a meal plan, we should first take one more step during the initial preparation phase – and this is to decide when you want to eat, as well as when you want to fast.

We are using the 16:8 intermittent fasting method in this book. This means that for eight hours every day, you will eat. The rest of the time, which includes a 16-hour period, you will be fasting. Even though this sounds simple enough, simply stating that you are following a 16:8 intermittent fasting plan does not give you a view on when exactly each of these windows should be. At what hour should you start to eat and at what hour should your fast period start?

There are different ways to implement this program – but do not try to split the eight hours up. You cannot allow yourself four hours of eating in the morning, fast until four in the afternoon, and then have another four-hour eating phase. This will not work and is not how the program is supposed to be initiated. Your eight hours should be straight up – a single session of eating that expands over an eight-hour period in total for every 24 hours that passes by.

I would suggest you ask yourself how important breakfast is to you. For some people, breakfast truly is the most effective meal of the day, but there are also many people who do not mind skipping breakfast. If you do feel that you are unable to go without breakfast, then you could think about starting your eating window in the morning when you get up.

I, on a personal note, do not recommend this. I have found that skipping breakfast and getting into your eating window later in the afternoon is a much better way of utilizing the benefits of intermittent fasting.

You might think that you won't be able to get through the morning and last until the late afternoon without a good breakfast, but you probably haven't given it a try with the intermittent fasting method in the past. I'm not saying it will be easy – you will need to get used to this new "tradition" – but if you can be patient and push through a little, you'll be able to reap the benefits.

If you find that you feel lethargic and experience fatigue during your mornings when you skip breakfast when you follow an intermittent fasting eating program, then pick up your favorite type of coffee when you go out to the supermarket again. Start your day with a freshly brewed cup of coffee – just be sure NOT to add any sugar, sweeteners, or milk. These will add calories and will essentially break your fast.

Many people find it hard to drink coffee without any creamer or sweetener. If this is you, don't worry – it just takes some getting used to. Plus, when you drink coffee like this, you'll start to experience a wide range of added benefits.

The caffeine in coffee is a natural stimulant. This means it will boost your cognitive function and help to avoid those moments of mental fatigue where all of your productivity goes out the window. You'll also experience a physical energy boost, which can really come in handy if you plan on doing your exercise routine early in the morning.

In addition to these potential benefits, a stimulant will also help to boost your metabolism. This means that you'll be able to experience a faster rate of fat burning when you decide to have a black, unsweetened cup of coffee to start your day. Plus, coffee has been linked to quite an impressive number of other health benefits that will surely simply add to your goal of living a healthier life.

At first, you might need to do some experimenting to find the right times that suit your lifestyle best, as well as satisfy your appetite more appropriately. I personally recommend that you start out with a plan where you break your fast at around four in the afternoon – you can then eat up until midnight, although most people go to bed way before then, so this is a very beneficial plan as you'll most likely shorten your eating window to around six hours.

If you would rather like to have breakfast, then you could opt for a program that lets you break your fast at around nine in the morning. You'll be able to eat until around five in the afternoon.

As I mentioned, these are not definite times that you MUST go with. Look at your schedule and consider your own lifestyle. The same timeframe for an eating window will not be ideal for everyone. You need to find what suits you best – you have eight hours to eat, just pick the right times that works best for you and fits in most appropriately with your schedule.

Calculate Your Ideal Daily Caloric Intake

Now we reach a very important part of your intermittent fasting program – calculating the most ideal number of calories that you should consume each day. In this step, it might also be a good idea to determine how many calories you'll have to burn. The data you calculate in this step will be crucial in the following section of the book, as you'll have to fit in various meals into your daily plan assure that your intake of calories is not too high, but rather fits into your daily caloric intake goal.

This is also a step that can be difficult since there are a lot of mixed opinions on how many calories you should consume each day and how you need to calculate your ideal caloric intake for specific goals that you are striving toward.

In most cases, men are advised to consume a higher number of calories each day than women. These are the general recommendations for maintaining your weight (taken you exercise enough to avoid a calorie surplus):

• Women: ~ 2,000 calories on a daily basis
• Men: ~ 2,500 calories on a daily basis

If 2,000 or 2,500 calories (depending on your gender, of course) is the recommended daily intake, then you would obviously have to lower this number in order to get to a daily caloric intake that will create a calorie deficit so that you can lose weight.

There are a number of factors that will have an impact on the actual recommended daily caloric intake that you should try to aim for. This includes:
• The current weight you are at
• Your age
• Your height
• Your current level of physical activity
• Your overall metabolic health

These are only some of the factors that will have an impact on your target daily calorie intake, as well as the calorie intake you should achieve to assist in reducing your body weight.

Let's say you are a woman and your goal is 2,000, then to create a calorie deficit to ensure weight loss can be possible, you'll need to bring it down to about 1,500 calories per day. Your physical activity should then be planned in such a way that it burns more than 1,500 calories on a day-to-day basis, which results in weight loss success.

If you want to be more specific, then consider using an online calorie requirement calculator. There are many free options available, and a simple Google search will give you some of the best ones on the first page's results.

Let's take a quick look at an example, just to help

you out and ensure you can better understand how the process works.

The dummy profile we will use is John Doe. He is 28 years old and male, measuring 1.6 meters. John currently weighs 103kg. His goal with an intermittent fasting plan is to lose fat, and his current activity level is light – he works in a place that requires him to be sedentary during the day, but he tries to be somewhat active when he is not at work.

To lose weight quickly, but still, in a safe way, John will have to reduce his daily caloric intake to around 1,505 calories.

Let's take a look at another example – Susan. Susan is a 35-year-old female, and she measures 1.5 meters. She weighs 115kg and wants to lose weight. With intermittent fasting on her side, Susan plans on becoming more active by implementing a range of intense exercise programs into her life, but her job still demands a more sedentary life at work.

To lose weight, Susan will need to adopt a diet plan that gives her around 1,684 calories each day.

As you can see, there is a lot of variables that come into play when calculating an ideal calorie intake number to target each day.

Another thing that I need you to note here is the fact that simply because this number is something you calculate does not mean it is a definite guide on how many calories you should consume every single day.

For most people, exercising every day can take up a lot of time and is not the ideal option. Most people will rather choose to include a more intense training session on fewer days of the week. You might, for example, choose to exercise on Mondays, Wednesdays, and Fridays.

When you do opt for a training program that has such a schedule, your intermittent fasting diet plan will need to be altered a little. On days where you will not be participating in these intense exercises, you will need to have a lower calorie intake. On days where you are going to be exercising a lot, however, you'll have to increase your calorie intake – this will help to ensure your body has adequate levels of "fuel" in order to continue working hard during your exercise protocols.

CHAPTER 6

CALORIE GOAL FORMULA

If you wish to get more technical and have some time on your hands to do a rather simple calculation, then I suggest you follow a specific formula in order to calculate a more accurate daily calorie goal. This will essentially be more useful than using generic advice.

To do this, you'll first calculate your BMR or your Basal Metabolic Rate. This is essentially the number of calories your body needs to survive in a resting state. You will then adjust the BMR according to your activity level, and then make another adjustment for the goal you are trying to achieve – which is to lose excess fat, in this case.

To do this, you'll have to determine your lean body mass and your fat percentage. To calculate your lean body mass, follow this formula: current weight – (current weight x (your current body fat percentage / 100). You'll then calculate your BMR with this formula: 370 + 21.6 x LBM (your Lean Body Mass that you calculated in the previous step.

Once you have your BMR, consider how active you are. If you are sedentary most of the time, then the formula is your BMR times 1.2. For light activity, BMR times 1.375. For moderate activity, BMR times 1.55. If you are very active, then BMR times 1.725.

All you need to do now is take your body fat percentage into account. If your body fat percentage is higher than 30%, then lower the number of calories calculated in the previous step by 30%. If you are between 20 and 30%, then lower calorie intake by 25%. For 10 to 20%, lower by 20%, and for those with a body fat percentage that is under 10%, lower your calorie intake by 15%.

The result is the number of calories you should ideally eat every day in order to ensure you can lose weight.

Sounds too complicated? Let's take a look at a quick example.

Let's call our sample person Joey. Joey weighs 120kg and has a body fat percentage of 32%. Joey only participates in light activities throughout the week.

Lean Body Mass: 120 − (120 x (32/100)) = 81.6
BMR: 370 + 21.6 x LBM = 2132
Activity adjustment: 2132 x 1.375 = 2931
Daily Calorie Recommendation: 2931 − 30% = 2052

Determine What Foods You Should Include In Your Meal Plan

Now that you have set up the appropriate calorie plan for yourself, it is time to move forward. You will now have to start setting up a food plan for yourself – but before we actually go into more detail in terms of the food plan or diet plan that you are going to be following for the next two weeks, let's first take a look at some of the most ideal foods that you should try to have in the meal plan you are planning to follow.

I'm not going to share a complete meal plan with you right this moment – we'll cover that in the next section. I just want to provide you with a few foods that are known to accelerate fat loss. These are the types of food that you should try to include in your diet in order to promote an improvement in your metabolism and to essentially help to speed up your weight loss results.

The foods I am about to share with you will not make up the entire diet plan that you will be following throughout the next two weeks while you implement intermittent fasting into your life. Instead, they will form somewhat of a basis or an outline for preparing meals. You'll still enjoy other types of food (not the fattening kind, however), and then add some of these foods to your meals to promote improvements in your efforts to lose weight.

Leafy Greens

Of course leafy green deserves its place at the top. Leafy greens include a range of different vegetables like collards, spinach, swiss chard, and kale. These are, without a doubt, some of the healthiest foods that you can eat, and they are excellent for anyone who is trying to shed some excess pounds.

The thing with leafy greens is these vegetables are very low in calories. They are also not loaded with carbohydrates like some vegetables and fruits are. On the other hand, leafy greens contain a lot of fiber, which is not only good for your digestive system but can also be an extremely useful tool in helping you shed those extra pounds that you had packed.

One scientific paper looked at numerous studies that have been conducted in the past and confirms that there is a positive relation between fiber intake and body weight. With a higher fiber intake, obesity can be prevented more effectively. Among people who are obese, an increase in fiber intake may yield a positive interaction with their body weight – both body fat and body weight tend to decrease among obese individuals who start to follow a high-fiber diet.

The paper explains that the primary mechanism in terms of how fiber assists in weight management lie with the ability of the substance to reduce appetite. When food intake is decreased through a higher fiber consumption, there are less excess calories in the body to be stored as fat at the end of the day.

Cruciferous Vegetables

Another class of vegetables that should definitely be included in your meal plan if you intend to lose weight would be cruciferous vegetables. These generally include Brussels sprouts, cabbage, broccoli, and cauliflower. All of these vegetables are also very good for your entire body and may yield positive results in terms of your weight loss efforts.

Cruciferous vegetables are, similar to leafy greens, loaded with high-quality plant-based fiber. This means that including more of these vegetables in your meal plan will help you feel fuller after you have had a meal. The end result is a decrease in your daily caloric intake.

In addition to being a great source of plant-based fibers, cruciferous vegetables can also help you increase your intake of protein, another important nutrient that is definitely crucial for any type of weight loss program.

A paper published in the American Journal of Clinical Nutrition explains that a diet that contains relatively high amounts of protein can be very effective in aiding a person in their weight loss program, and can also be an effective mechanism for weight management in general.

The study explains that protein intake should be equal to around 1.2 to 1.6 grams of protein per one kilogram of body weight, with an approximate minimum protein per meal suggested to be around 25 grams. In turn, this amount of protein can assist in various elements that are related to weight management, including:

- Appetite will be reduced and, in turn, lead to a lowering of the daily caloric intake
- Risk factors associated with cardiometabolic health are improved
- Body fat can be reduced when combined with an appropriate meal plan and, of course, a physical activity program

A Boiled Potato

Potatoes are often thought to be a bad food when it comes to weight loss, but when used the right way, a simple boiled potato can actually help you reach your weight loss goals. The important thing to do here is to boil the potato and then allow it to cool for some time before you consume it.

When a boiled potato cools down, it leads to the formation of a type of substance known as resistant starch. This is similar to fiber and will be able to improve your satiety – that said, you'll feel full for some time, allowing you to get through your day without opting for foods that will simply add to your calories and cause weight gain.

One medium sized potato contains around 163 calories, which means you will still have a significant amount of calories to play with during the rest of your day and it will fit in perfectly with your daily meal plan.

In addition to the resistant starch that forms when you boil a potato and allow it to cool for a few minutes, this food is also packed with an impressive variety of nutrients. Thus, you'll also be giving your body a good dose of essential vitamins and minerals, while also satisfying your appetite at the same time.

A potato will give you vitamin C, calcium, iron, and there are two grams of fiber in a medium-sized potato – this is excluding the resistant starch that will be formed when you cool down a boiled potato.

The phytonutrients found in potato will further benefit you, and there are antioxidants that can help to fight against free radicals in your body, promoting heart and brain health, while also fighting against cancer and many other diseases.

CHAPTER 7

INTERMITTENT FASTING MEALS

Now that we have gone through all of the most crucial steps that need to be taken and, of course, thoroughly understood in order to adopt an intermittent fasting meal plan that will help you lose weight, it is time that you look at a simple two-week plan that you can use to kickstart your journey.

There are many diets out there that can essentially be followed. It is, however, very beneficial if you take your own particular daily caloric requirements for weight loss into account, and consider any type of condition that you have – these would include food sensitivities, allergies, and intolerances – in order to develop a meal plan that is ideally suited to your unique body.

Still, you can take an existing meal plan, follow it, and then make adjustments as you go in order to suit better your specific circumstances – adjust according to your body weight, goal, and food preferences.

As I promised earlier in this book, I will now be sharing a basic meal plan with you, and I'll include a list of useful and delicious recipes with you.

This is how it is going to work. I'll first share with you a basic overview of a specific plan that you should be following for the next 14 days (two weeks in total). I'll tell you how to adjust your calories every day, when to eat, when to fast, etc.

After I shared the plan with you, I will share a large list of great weight-loss-friendly recipes with you. Each recipe will be accompanied by details such as how many calories the meal has. You will then be able to go through your daily plan and decide each day which particular recipe you wish to try out.

There might be times when you will have to make some adjustments to the recipes that I have shared – remember that you worked out your daily caloric goal before. It really is impossible to specify hundreds of different scenarios that may apply now. Thus, take the meal plan and even the recipes I offer you here as a guideline – then adjust them according to the previous steps that we went through.

From this point on, we'll be focusing on an example person in order to simplify things. We'll consider a man with an ideal daily caloric intake of 2500 calories, and a modified goal caloric intake for weight loss of 2000 calories. With this reduction in calories, weight loss will not happen overnight. In fact, you might not even experience significant results within the first week – but I really urge you to continue following the diet and implementing the steps I share with you.

It is better to lose weight gradually than too quickly. Gradual weight loss usually provides for a safer process of reducing your body weight, reduces the risk of suffering from poor nutrition while you are dieting, and also yields longer term results. This means you'll be able to shed those excess pounds that you need to get rid of and then keep them off because you have adopted healthier habits, instead of jumping from one fad diet to the next one.

CHAPTER 8

TWO-WEEK INTERMITTENT FASTING MEAL PLAN

Before we take a look at a meal plan that you can use for the next two weeks to help you get started with intermittent fasting, I want first to advise you to consider the fact that we looked at a schedule earlier in this guide. I explained how you will need to decide when you would like to have your eating windows, and when you would like to fast. The decisions you made at this point in the book will now come into play.

While I will be providing a basic overview of a meal schedule that you can follow in order for you to be able to take full advantage of intermittent fasting, you will need to take the specific schedule that you decided on earlier into account here.

I personally prefer to fast during the morning and to skip breakfast. This helps to keep my body in a fat burning mode while I get my day started – I do, however, enjoy a cup of coffee (without sugar and creamer, of course).

Thus, the plan that I will be providing you with below is basically how I personally follow the intermittent fasting eating plan. You can use the plan exactly as I give it to you here, or you can make appropriate adjustments that will better suit the schedule you wish to follow – according to when you wish to implement your eating window and when you would like to fast during this eating plan.

Another thing that I would like you to note before we get set on this program is the fact that you will have further modifications in your daily caloric intake, which will essentially depend on whether you will have a resting day or an active day.

Without further delay, let's dive into the two-week program that I promised you earlier on.

Day 1:

Day type: resting day
Calorie intake: 1600 calories

Your first day will likely be the most difficult. You'll feel hungry when you first get started. Remember that your body has not yet adapted to the intermittent fasting program that you are now following, so give it time. It is, however, crucial that you avoid giving in to those temptations – which will haunt you today!

Everyone wakes up at a different time, but as I suggested, I'm taking a lot from my own schedule here, so let's get started with day one.

07:00 -> Wake up, prepare yourself a delicious cup of coffee. Use your favorite blend of coffee. Just the coffee and some boiling water – remember that sugar and creamer are both no-nos.

10:30 -> You're probably starting to feel some hunger coming on now. Don't worry, and it's your first day. If you see a box of donuts laying around, do NOT give in to the temptation. Be patient. Have a glass of water. Continue to have water as the day goes by, every time that you feel hungry.

14:00 -> You're doing great if you're still holding up. Grab yourself a bottle of sparkling water, no added flavoring agents or sugars, please. Drink up to get past the last hour.

15:00 -> Congrats! You've reached the time to break your fast. Now, we're going at it slow. You've been fasting all day long now, so you don't want to overload your digestive system. Have a healthy snack – take a look at the granola bar recipe I share in the next section. The bar is delicious and low in calories. Try to stay under 300 calories for this meal.

18:00 -> Time for that second meal of the day. We're still keeping it a little low and waiting for a bigger feast that will come later tonight. Have a medium-sized meal that counts to about 500 calories in total. There are various options that you can enjoy now – again, take a look at the recipes I have shared to get an idea of what you can prepare. If you like one of the low-calorie options, but the calorie count is significantly low, see if you can double the portion size to reach 500.

22:00 -> At about 10, you should have your biggest meal of the day. For today, limit your calorie intake to 800 with this meal. Remember that it's a resting day, so you don't need excess calories to make up for the calories that you burnt during exercise – since you didn't exercise, of course.

Day 2:

Day type: active
Calorie intake: 2400 calories

Today, we're stepping up our game and adding in some physical activity to burn some calories. You're boosting your calorie intake for the day in order to ensure you will have enough strength and energy to keep up with the demands of physical exercise.

Let's get this day going!

06:30 -> We're getting up earlier today to make some time for a session of physical activity. Let's get the day going with some coffee again – that will help to give you that initial boost you need for exercise.

07:00 -> Time for some exercise. There are so many activities you can participate in. For today, we're not going to be too intense. Let's do some jogging. Take a jog for about 15 to 20 minutes. Once you get home and you have some strength left, pick up some weights and start a session of strength training exercises. If you don't have weight, fall down onto the floor and do some push-ups, as well as a couple of sit-ups. Remember to stay hydrated while you are exercising – have a big glass of water to finish off the session.

10:30 -> Let's do another glass of water just to help reduce your hunger and make you feel full.

14:00 -> Just like yesterday, we'll do another bottle of sparkling water now. We are going to push things one hour further today – your first meal will not be at 3 pm, but rather at 4 pm.

16:00 -> Time has arrived for that first meal. We'll start off with a bigger meal than yesterday, but still small enough not to overload your system. Opt for something that gives you about 500 calories.

19:00 -> The second meal of the day is here – with this, be creative, but don't exceed 700 calories in total.

22:00 -> Again the final meal of the day, the biggest feast that you are going to be enjoying. I suggest limiting yourself to about 1200 calories for this meal. You can go a little lower if you are concerned about the meal being too big before you go to sleep, but avoid going below the 900 marks, just so that you still get more calories than yesterday to make up for the calories that you burnt this morning.

Day 3 to 21

I've given you an example of how a day should go when you are not going to exercise, as well as on your physically active days. Now, you can follow the same example for the next few days until you reach day 21.

The details I just gave you lay out a solid foundation for a very (VERY) effective intermittent fasting program that focuses on giving you an appropriate eating window, while also allowing you to fast for an appropriate period of time to ensure you can thoroughly experience the benefits that intermittent fasting has for you.

From here on out, you'll need to start experimenting a little. If you feel that 4 pm in the afternoon is too long to wait for a meal, then narrow the window and have your first meal at 3 pm. It is important that you don't eat too frequently, however. Don't have a meal every hour and divide your calories up into eight different meals. Instead, have three meals and perhaps work in a couple of snacks between these meals – as long as they fit into your daily calorie allowance.

On days where you will be physically active, you have a larger number of calories to play with. In these cases, you are able to work in some extra snacks, for example. Let's say between your second and third meal, at around eight or nine at night, and you can select to have a small snack or a very small meal of just a few calories (maybe 200 calories, for example).

As I mentioned before, be sure to check out the granola bar I share below – I personally make these once a week – about five at a time – and then space them out as snacks throughout my days.

Another tip – for some people, having a heavy meal just before they go to bed is too much. It can sometimes make you feel uncomfortable. Every person is different. For me – I really enjoy having my feast meal at the end of the day, rewarding myself for holding out the entire day and building up my hunger for that awesome meal.

For others, however, an adjustment may be needed. If this is your case, then consider making the second meal, which you should have between six and seven ideally, your feast meal. Add the majority of your calories here, and then have a smaller meal at night.

If you still feel that you do not want to eat so late at night, just before you get into bed, then you might also consider moving your eating window a little down the line and breaking your fast a little earlier in the day. For example, you could have your first meal at one in the afternoon. This way, you will eat your second meal at approximately three to four, and finish your eating window at around seven or eight, instead of at ten.

Just be sure to take my advice about your first

meal into account – try not to overload on calories when you first break the first. This will be heavy on your stomach, and it can lead to discomfort.

CHAPTER 9

WEIGHT LOSS RECIPES FOR YOUR INTERMITTENT FASTING PROGRAM

We've looked at a great two-week meal plan program that you can follow, so now it is time that we consider some recipes that you can prepare for yourself on this particular meal plan. Now, the recipes that I share with you below can be used as different meals to fill in the meal plan that you are going to be following.

What I need you to do is thoroughly consider each of these recipes – especially take a look at the calories of each recipe that I share with you. This will give you a good idea of when you should have this meal and how much of an impact it will have on the number of calories that you can consume during the day.

This is also where you can get creative. You can mix

and match. You choose what you want to eat – and you'll discover in just a moment that reducing your daily caloric intake does not mean you have to eat a bowl of salad every day. There are many delicious meals that you can prepare that are low in calories, yet high in nutrients.

Home-Made Granola Bars

So, I really like to break my fast with something that is yummy, yet does not expose my body to sugars and other unhealthy ingredients. At the same time, I also do not like to break my fast with something heavy that is going to overload my stomach and my digestive system. I have been fasting for 16 hours – so I prefer to go in slowly. This is why I really love these home-made granola bars. They are nutritious and really good for you, and they are relatively low in calories.

The recipe that I am about to share with you will yield 10 bars in total. This is a great bar to make upfront and then store them in an airtight container – don't overload yourself on them. Instead, pack one in your bag every day just to break your fast without overdoing it.

Each of these bars contains about 238 calories, which will not cut in too deep into your daily caloric allowance. Each bar is also filled with 6.2 grams of fiber, 6.8 grams of protein, and about nine grams of fat.

The ingredients you will need include:

- Half a cup of raw almonds. Be sure to chop them up roughly. For an alternative version, using pecan nuts or walnuts instead.
- Two tablespoons of chia seeds.
- Two tablespoons of flax seeds.

- Two tablespoons of sunflower seeds.
- Quarter-cup peanut butter. It is best to opt for an organic peanut butter. Alternatively, you can use almond butter.
- Two tablespoons of hemp seeds
- One-and-a-half cup of oats (rolled and preferably the gluten-free kind, if possible)
- A heaped cup of dates
- About quarter-cup of a sweetening agent. You can use honey preferably, but maple syrup or agave nectar can also work great.

I sometimes add a couple of banana chips and some additional nuts to my granola bars, but remember that this also adds more calories, so be careful.

To make these homemade granola bars, simply follow these instructions:

1. Start by turning on the oven to about 180-degrees Celsius and then toast both the almonds (or another type of nut that you chopped), along with the oats, for a maximum of 15 minutes.
2. You need to cut the dates up into very small pieces, preferably by using a food processor. If you do not own a food processor, then try to cut it with a knife as small as you possibly can.
3. Now mix the seeds, the oats, the dates, and the almonds in one bowl.
4. Place the sweetening agent, such as agave nectar

or honey, that you chose into a saucepan. Be sure to turn the stove top up to a low heat setting to avoid burning the mixture. Add the peanut butter. Once the mixture is warm and starts to combine, stir it once or twice and then pour the mixture over the seeds and oats mixture that you previously combined. Thoroughly mix the combination that is now in your mixing bowl.

5. Now, simply transfer this combination of ingredients to an appropriate dish, cover the dish with some plastic wrap. Be sure to squeeze down on the mixture that is now in the dish in order to compress them.

6. Allow the mixture to cool in the freezer for about 20 minutes. Remove and then cut it up into 10 bars of equal size.

That's it. Be sure to keep one with you to have when the time comes to break your fast and enter your eating window if this is something that you like and prefer.

Pork Tenderloin with Some Veggies

If you are looking for a quick and easy recipe that you can have, let's say as your last meal of the day, then some pork tenderloin, along with some veggies, maybe a great option for you. This entire meal contains less than 800 calories per serving, which means it is a great way to keep your calories low while still having a great meal.

Each serving will contain approximately 740 calories, to be more specific.

The ingredients that you will need in order to prepare this meal include:

• Approximately 220 grams of pork tenderloin. This will likely equal two pieces at most.
• About four tablespoons of almonds. Slice the almonds so that it is easier to prepare your meal.
• Two cups of green beans, preferably steamed.
• Up to two sweet potatoes.

Your pork should simply be seasoned with some pepper and salt. You should add it to a skillet and then place the pork chops in the oven at about 220 degrees Celsius. Leave the pork in the heated oven for about 15 minutes.

Slice the tenderloin into smaller slices. Serve it up with the green beans and up to two baked sweet potatoes.

Broccoli Soup with Cheese and Chicken

Remember we previously discussed the many health benefits associated with broccoli? Well, this is a creative recipe that gives you the benefits of this great vegetable, along with the added protein-boosting advantages of chicken. Plus, the meal is truly delicious and can be a great second meal of the day.

Each serving of this meal will give you about 360 calories. This is a very low amount of calories, so it can fit in great with your daily meal plan.

Let's take a look at the ingredients you need:

- About a cup of broccoli, chopped into pieces.
- About a cup of parsnips, also chopped into pieces.
- Quarter-cup shredded cheddar cheese, low-fat option preferably to keep calories low.
- A small chicken breast, about 110 to 120 grams.
- Quarter-cup of chicken stock, preferably a low-fat option as well.
- One tablespoon of almonds, sliced into smaller pieces
- A teaspoon of lemon juice

Along with these ingredients, you will also need some pepper and salt to season the chicken.

To make this recipe, simply follow these instructions:

1. Steam together the parsnips and the broccoli
2. While the veggies are steaming, bake the chicken in the oven
3. After steaming, add the cheddar cheese and the chicken stock
4. Use a food processor or another appropriate kitchen appliance to puree this mixture
5. Sprinkle some of the chopped almonds over the mixture
6. Sprinkle some lemon juice, pepper, and salt on the chicken
7. Serve up and enjoy

Gazpacho, Chicken, And Some Lemon Slices

This is really one of my favorite meals – it combines a range of delicious ingredients in one meal, and it is still relatively low in calories. Whenever I decide to prepare this particular dish, I would usually either use it as my second (middle) meal, or I would add another chicken breast to up the calorie intake for my feast meal at the end of the day.

Each serving of this meal gives you 414 calories. You can experiment by making a double serving of the entire meal, or perhaps by adding another chicken breast. If you prefer, you can add another vegetable or two as well. Just be sure to calculate the additional calories that you are adding to your meal when you decide to make an adjustment to this recipe.

Let's start with the ingredients for the chicken:

- 100g chicken breast
- One tablespoon olive oil
- One teaspoon rosemary, fresh preferably
- Half a lemon – cut the lemon into slices

All you need to do is use a brush to pain the olive oil over the chicken. Add the rosemary, along with the lemon slices, on top of the chicken. Add the chicken breast to your oven – bake at about 180 degrees Celsius for approximately half an hour.

And now, for the Gazpacho – these are the ingredients that you will need:

- About three cloves of garlic – cut them into small pieces or mince them using a food processor
- A quarter-cup chopped cucumber
- About one tablespoon vinegar, preferably white wine vinegar
- A cup of tomatoes, stewed
- About half a cup of chopped onions
- A quarter-cup of chopped green pepper

Making the Gazpacho is quick and easy. Simply add all of these ingredients to your blender and hit the start button. Wait for the combo to blend and mix properly, and then serve this with the chicken.

Shrimp Paste and Salad

Even though pasta is definitely not considered the best choice of food for people who are looking to lose weight, you can still add a delicious pasta-based meal to your daily diet and still have a calorie deficit. The important part here is to be wary of how much pasta you eat and what other ingredients your meal contains. This shrimp pasta and salad is a really delicious meal that you can enjoy at any time. It has a moderate amount of calories, with each serving giving you about 465 calories. If you feel that you want to feast on this meal, then double it up for a 930 dosing of calories – this can easily make up your big meal for the day while being delicious and also good for you at the same time.

The main ingredients that you will need for this recipe include:

- Approximately 85 grams of poached shrimp
- Half a cup of dry rigatoni – cook this up according to the instructions provided on the packaging of the pasta
- Half a tablespoon of pine nuts
- Three black olives, you can opt for large ones, and be sure to slice them up
- Two teaspoons of grated Parmesan cheese
- Half a cup of sun-dried tomatoes, be sure to drain the packaging and then puree them using a food processor

You will also need a few extra ingredients to make the salad. These include:

- A quarter cup of tomatoes, chopped
- Half a tablespoon of balsamic vinegar
- One cup romaine lettuce
- Half a cup of cucumber slices

The salad is easy to prepare. Simply mix all of the ingredients in a bowl, and you're ready to go. For the pasta, toss together the pasta with all the other ingredients.

As you can see, this is an exceptionally easy meal to prepare and also very fast – you simply cook up some pasta, poach a couple of shrimps, toss them together, prepare a side salad, and you're ready to eat up.

Meatballs with Spaghetti

Ah, yes, this one is truly one of my favorites – mainly because it gives you a good dose of both fiber and protein, two essentials of any type of weight loss plan that will yield successful results. Plus, this is a truly delicious meal. I usually prepare a single serving on my rest days, but when I am on a training day, I sometimes up the recipe three times, giving me a meal that is very close to a thousand calories – this way, I can ensure that my muscles gain enough protein and other nutrients in order to heal from a hard day at the gym.

Be prepared as this one takes a little more time than simply tossing together some pasta and other ingredients – you'll have to make the meatballs yourself. On the other hand, it's always fun to set aside some time to spend in the kitchen. Isn't it satisfying to know exactly what you put into your meals?

This meal contains 330 calories per serving. If you up it by three, then you get a meal with a 990 serving of calories.

To prepare a plate of meatballs and spaghetti, you will need the following ingredients:

- Quarter cup of spinach leaves
- One sweet potato
- Quarter teaspoon of oregano

- Quarter cup of farro, cooked
- One tablespoon of onion, chopped
- One egg whites
- Quarter teaspoon turmeric
- A pinch of both pepper and salt
- About 115 grams of ground turkey (it might sound like a lot, but this is still a very low-calorie option)
- Approximately one tablespoon of Asiago cheese, grated

That is all the ingredients you need – now, on to the actual recipe to get you going...

Before you get started, be sure to preheat your oven. You do not want to place your meatballs into a cold oven – your oven should be hot so that you can time your meatballs correctly. Set the oven to about 180 degrees Celsius.

On to the steps:

1. Mix together (by hand) the ground turkey, spinach leaves, egg whites, turmeric, pepper, salt, oregano, farro, and, of course, the onion.
2. After thoroughly mixing the ingredients by hand, divide the mixture into four parts and then roll each of these parts into balls. They should have a diameter of approximately one inch.
3. Line a pan with some parchment paper and place the balls on the paper, spreading them out evenly. Place the pan inside the oven and let

them bake for approximately half an hour. Make sure they are golden brown before you remove them.

4. While the meatballs are in the oven, wash the sweet potatoes and then peel them. After peeling them, use the peeler to create ribbons from the sweet potato's flesh. Place these ribbons into boiling water with a pinch of salt, and then drain them properly.

5. Once the meatballs are done baking, remove them from the oven.

6. Serve up the meatballs with the sweet potato ribbons, as well as some Asiago cheese sprinkled on the top.

Roasted Vegetables with Rosemary and Serrano Ham

Next up let's take a look at a great recipe for those who really enjoy digging into a plate of vegetables. There's some meat, too, however, so if you do want a meaty taste with your meal, don't worry.
This roasted veggies dish is low in calories and contains a high amount of protein, as well as fiber. This will definitely come in handy in your weight loss efforts, keep you full for longer, and be a real benefit to your digestive system.

Each serving gives you about 322 calories. You'll get about 21 grams of protein and 10 grams of fiber per serving.

The ingredients for this roasted vegetables with rosemary and serrano ham dish include the following:

- One tablespoon of sherry vinegar
- Two teaspoons of olive oil
- Two teaspoons of rosemary, fresh and chopped up
- About 220 grams of asparagus, be sure to trim the asparagus and cut them into small pieces
- About 220 grams of Brussel sprouts, choose small ones and chop them in half
- Two tablespoons of manchego cheese shaved
- About 30 grams of Serrano ham, tear the ham

into small pieces

Now that you have the ingredients turn the stove on to about 220 degrees Celsius. Your oven should ideally be preheated so that you can simply pop the dish into the oven when ready and get going.

Let's get started with the dish. Get out a baking sheet – now add the asparagus and the Brussels sprouts. Sprinkle over the oil, the rosemary, and some black pepper if you have any available. Place the baking sheet in the oven and let them roast. Be sure to stir the veggie mixture once while it is still in the oven.

Once roasted, mix in the vinegar, as well as the ham. Place the baking tray back into the oven for a minute or two. When serving up, be sure to sprinkle some of the manchego cheese on top of the dish.

Butternut Squash Soup with some Beef Stir-Fry

For many people, a true balance meal should include both veggies and some meat. This is great as it gives you the benefits of both food types. We're getting a little creative here by introducing some solid meat to the plate, along with a veggie soup.

This is a very easy meal to prepare, and it is also low in calories. Each serving gives you about 450 calories.

Let's start with the ingredients. To prepare this meal, you will need the following ingredients:

- Half a cup of shiitake mushrooms, slice them to be prepared.
- About two teaspoons of olive oil.
- Approximately 85 grams of tenderloin fillet steak. Be sure to slice the steak into thin slices. You can, of course, increase how much steak you add to increase the calories of the meal, making this a great choice for your daily feast meal.
- Half an onion. Slice the onion into rings.
- About half a cup of bulgur, cooked, of course

In addition to all of the above-mentioned ingredients, you'll also need some butternut squash soup. You could opt to make this yourself, but that will simply add more time to preparing dinner.

Instead, it might be a good idea to buy a pre-made butternut soup. If you do choose this route, then you should try to opt for a low-sodium option and see if you can find an organic butternut squash soup. To prepare the beef, stir fry the steak slices, along with the mushroom and the onion. Use the olive oil to stir-fry these ingredients.

When serving up, start with the bulgur. Thereafter, add the beef stir-fry on top of the bulgur. Finally, don't forget to serve up with the butternut soup. You might want to heat up the butternut soup before serving.

Lemon, Dill, And Salmon

Next up is a very low-calorie meal that is perfect if you want to start the day slow, but you do want to opt for a meal instead of just a granola bar or another snack-based meal. This is a delicious meal and gives you a healthy dose of salmon, a type of fish that is known to be high in essential fatty acids, such as omega-3 fatty acids. This is good for heart health, for improving cholesterol levels, and for better brain health.

A single serving of this dish gives you about 261 calories. This means if you do decide to include this one, you will still have quite a lot of additional calories that you can play with during the rest of the day.

To prepare the dish, you will need the following ingredients:

- One teaspoon of dill
- About three-quarter cup of parsnips
- One tablespoon of lemon juice
- One and a half cup of broccoli – chop up the broccoli and steam it
- Approximately 140 grams of salmon, preferably a wild-caught type

Making this dish is really easy. Simply add the salmon to a dish and sprinkle with the dill and the lemon juice. You should preferably bake this dish at a low heat – about 110 degrees Celsius. Be sure to preheat the oven before placing in the baking dish. Now, once the oven is heated, add the baking tray with the salmon for approximately 15 minutes.

Pesto Pasta

The next one on our list is a delicious pasta dish that has just over 400 calories and contains a good combination of meat and veggies to help you load up on healthy nutrients. Similar to the other recipes, this one can easily be doubled in order to increase the calorie content and make it an ideal choice for feasting on those training days.

You only need a few ingredients for this one, including:

- One-third cup of chicken breast – dice the chicken breast into somewhat small pieces
- About one-third cup of green beans – cook the beans beforehand
- A couple of cherry tomatoes, cut into halves
- A cup of linguine – cook this beforehand as well
- Approximately one-quarter cup of pesto sauce
- A quarter cup of Parmesan, shredded
- A pinch of both pepper and salt

Now that you have collected all of the ingredients, let's take a look at the simple steps needed to prepare this great meal:

1. Get a bowl and combine the diced chicken breast, the green beans (pre-cooked, the tomatoes, salt, and pepper, as well as the pesto sauce.)

2. Now, add the linguine to your mixture.
3. Finally, when serving up this meal, sprinkle with some of the Parmesan cheese

Quinoa with Zesty Tofu

Looking for something that is low in calories, great for your digestive system, and something different? Then try out this great quinoa dish, served with some tofu. You only need a few ingredients and preparing the meal is exceptionally easy. This meal gives you about 320 calories per serving.

Here's a list of the ingredients you need:

- One teaspoon cilantro
- One cup quinoa – pre-cook the quinoa
- About two tablespoons of avocado dices
- Three tablespoons worth of red pepper, diced
- Approximately 50 grams of tofu, choose the extra-firm kind and chop into cubes
- Two teaspoons of lime juice, preferably from a fresh lime

There are no special or complex instructions for preparing this meal. Simply combine all of the ingredients that I listed above, serve up, and enjoy.

Summer Farrotto

The last recipe I'd like to share here is another great choice as it combines healthy ingredients, along with useful fiber, and it is still a low-calorie option that can easily be adjusted to make up for the calories you still need to fill up for the day. This one, however, is higher in calories than some of the other options we have tried – doubling up on this particular recipe is really great if you need to load up after you have had a rough day at the gym, or even when you still need to go to the gym.

To prepare this delicious, yet low-calorie summer farrotto, you need these ingredients:

- One cup of yellow squash, diced
- One chicken breast, boneless and skinless, about 85 grams
- Quarter cup of red onion, sliced
- Half a cup of farro, dry
- One tablespoon of Parmesan cheese, grated
- One tablespoon of parsley, chopped
- Two tablespoons of olive oil – divide in two

After collecting all the ingredients, let's start the process of preparing the meal:

1. Start by using one tablespoon olive oil to sear the chicken in the pan. Add some pepper, as well as salt, to the chicken.

2. Dice up the chicken into smaller pieces.
3. With the oil still remaining in the pan, add the squash and onion, saute' these two ingredients.
4. Add the Farro and make sure it gets coated in the oil that was added previously.
5. Now, add about two-thirds of cup water to the mixture and allow the mixture to start boiling.
6. Once the mixture boils, stir once and then reduce the heat of the stove. Cover the mixture with a lid and allow to cook for approximately 20 minutes.
7. After 20 minutes, stir in the parsley, as well as the parmesan cheese and the chicken.
8. Serve up and enjoy.

CHAPTER 10

EXTRA TIPS TO GET THE MOST OUT OF INTERMITTENT FASTING

Congratulations on reaching this part of the book. If you have followed through up until this point, then you should know by now just how beneficial intermittent fasting can be – you might have already started to implement the strategies and recipes that I have shared with you. If so, then good for you. You are on your way to a better and healthier life, a lower body weight, a better body composition, and let's not forget a reduced risk of many diseases.

Before we finish off with this book, however, I do have a few final tips that I would like to share with you. The information I have provided here are already invaluable because they will put you on the right path to lose weight successfully through both diet and the intermittent fasting program – but what

I am about to share with you will ultimately help to speed up your results and give you an even greater goal to look forward to.

Adjust Your Diet Plan as You Go

I shared an excellent diet plan with you in this book, and it is perfectly normal and okay to follow the plan for the full two weeks that I have designed it for. Even after that, you may continue with the program in order to experience more benefits, such as reduced body weight and to gain an improvement in your overall health.

Now, at the same time, I do want to note that following one single plan over an extended period of time will often not offer you the best results that you could achieve through intermittent fasting.

The thing is every person is different – you are unique. For this reason, a specific meal plan that works for you will likely not be ideal for every single person.

This means that the diet program that I introduced you in this book might be able to work, but you may need to make some modifications as you go along in order to achieve the specific goals that you have in mind with the program that you are implementing.

Sure, you are not a dietician with years of experience in the industry, which really does make it somewhat harder for you to develop an appropriate diet plan that will suit you and help you achieve the goals you are striving toward. This, however, does not necessarily mean that it will be impossible for you to make simple adjustments in order to reach those weight loss goals.

Here's an example: you follow the diet plan that I have provided you here to the point, and prepare the specific meals that I have provided you with. Even though you implement these meal plans every day and you avoid binge eating, you find that you are not losing a lot of weight. In this case, there might not be an appropriate caloric deficit in your weight management plan.

When a caloric deficit is not present, it means you won't be able to lose weight – we have covered this already in a previous chapter in the book. If this is the case with you, then it means you will need to adjust your diet to reduce your daily caloric intake. This will essentially improve your caloric deficit and ensure you can lose weight more effectively through your intermittent fasting weight loss plan.

Don't Overlook The Importance Of Exercise In a Weight Loss Strategy

I have seen a lot of people start with an intermittent fasting plan and end up complaining that the program is not working for them. The same person would then tell me that they do not have a very physical lifestyle.

You should have read the topic where I explained how intermittent fasting is used for weight loss already by now, so you should understand that without expending calories each day, you won't be able to lose that excess fat that has accumulated inside your body.

Expending calories mean being physically active. Unfortunately, quite a large percentage of the worldwide population are living sedentary lifestyles. With a sedentary lifestyle, you are really "paving the way" for weight gain. If you are not physically active, you won't be able to burn an adequate number of calories each day for weight loss to be possible in the first place.

Thus, when you decide to follow my intermittent fasting weight loss cookbook and meal plan, then you should be sure also to include an appropriate exercise plan. Make sure you are physically active according to the prescribed standards – you should be physically active on a few days each week at a minimum.

The more you exercise, the more calories you will burn, of course. At the same time, you should be sure not to overdo things in terms of physical activity. There really is no use in causing yourself injury due to overtraining – this will only lead to temporary disability and will make training harder for the next few days (sometimes weeks or months if you suffer a more serious injury).

It is best to create a balanced exercise plan for yourself and then test it out. Listen to your body and understand when you are pushing yourself, as well as when you have some extra capacity available to up your game at the gym.

You will have to take your daily calorie consumption into account here – we did discuss how you can calculate your ideal daily calorie requirement in a previous section. This data will definitely come in handy here. Calculate an appropriate exercise plan that will ensure your daily caloric expenditure reached through physical exercise will reach past your daily caloric intake.

Deal with Hunger Pangs Like a Boss

Let's tackle a topic that you will likely face yourself. Hunger pangs are something that we all experience when we first start out with an intermittent fasting plan. You suddenly have to get your body adjusted to an entirely new way of eating. No longer do you get up in the morning and cook up some eggs and bacon. You have to get up and drink water, or perhaps have a cup of coffee, but you'll have to wait until the afternoon before you get to have your first meal.

So, the question now is, should you give in to the temptations that you will be experiencing, especially during those first few days, or should you implement an appropriate strategy to help you better cope with these hunger pangs and the cravings that you are going to experience.

There are different strategies that you can use to cope with your cravings. One would be to drink a glass of water if you feel hungry and you can feel those cravings building up. This is an effective strategy for lots of people, but not for everyone, of course. If you find that plain water or even filtered water does not work well for you, then I suggest you try some fizzy water (carbonated water). Be sure not to opt for carbonated water with added sweetening agents, as these are loaded with some carbs. Rather just opt for plain sparkling water. The carbonation in the water can help to make you feel full for a while to ensure you can get through to your eating window without giving in to your temptations.

It is important that you are patient and practice self-control when cravings start building up. Giving in to these cravings should not be considered okay now-and-then, as this will break the fasting window and it will yield less effective results compared to ensuring you last until you are inside of your eating window.

Avoid Eating These Foods

With intermittent fasting, a lot of people tend to follow their usual eating habits in terms of the specific foods that they put on their plate during each meal, expecting that they will lose weight just because they have fasted during the morning, night, and a part of the afternoon.

While intermittent fasting may help to improve metabolism and support digestive function that will ultimately improve your ability to lose weight, the food you eat still counts. As you might have noted, the meal plans that I shared with you in this cookbook generally combines a range of healthy foods in order to ensure you get the nutrients you need without loading up on too many carbs. I did include a lot of delicious options that you can try out.

Just as there are a lot of foods that you can surely include in your diet to help you lose that extra weight that is causing you concern, there are also some foods that you should always try to avoid if your goal is to lose weight.

Below, I would like to share some of the most important foods that you should try to exclude from your diet in order to improve the results you are able to achieve when you implement the recipes and meal plans I have provided you within this book.

- Fried foods, of course, should be at the top of my list. There is no doubt that fried foods are one particularly common reason for the world to be so obese. Millions of people eat fried foods as much as every day. This does not only cause them to gain in weight, but also to experience a rise in cholesterol levels, be at a higher risk of heart disease, and more.
- Fast foods, along with fried foods, since most chains that offer fast foods tend to deep fry their food in the worst types of oil and fat to make them more 'tasty' for the general public. Unfortunately, this also adds more fat to your belly, thighs, arms, and other areas of your body.
- Corn is another food that really isn't the best

choice for people who are trying to lose weight. Sure, it is not an unhealthy food, but consider the fact that this is a type of grain that is relatively high in sugar. The sugar spike experienced when you eat corn leads to the release of insulin, triggering inflammation and taking you one step closer to the dreadful complications of insulin resistance.

In addition to all of these, be sure to be wary of added sugars in everything you eat. For example, if you visit your local supermarket and grab a healthy bar to use as the food to break your fast, the fact that the word "healthy" appears on the bar does not necessarily mean it is truly healthy.

Always look at the ingredients of what you buy and what you will be putting into your body. Making your own healthy energy bars at home might be a better solution as well.

CHAPTER 11

CONCLUSION

Whether you are only overweight or have already reached the point where you are considered obese, excess weight in the body can lead to a number of adverse health effects that can eventually cause life-threatening conditions to develop. When excess fat accumulates, weight loss becomes a crucial component of improving health and ultimately extending a person's lifespan.

There are different strategies that you can use, and we focused on one particularly popular option in this book – intermittent fasting. In particular, we looked at how you can use the 16:8 intermittent fasting technique to help you shed excess body fat, while also building lean muscle mass and improving your overall body composition.

In addition to telling you how you can use the 16:8 intermittent fasting technique for weight loss, I also shared some highly effective and delicious meal options that you can use to ensure you can lose weight successfully while following this particular method of intermittent fasting.

From here, you can start to experiment with the meals that you include in your daily diet. There really is no one-size-fits-all option when it comes to including a specific meal plan in your intermittent fasting plan. The guidance I provided you with here will help you better realize how you should get started.

Once you implement the meal plan that I discussed with you here, you should already be able to start experiencing the benefits that are associated with intermittent fasting. After a week or two, you'll be able to see if the diet helps you lose weight and make appropriate adjustments to the meal plan that you are following to better suit your needs, as well as the specific goals that you have in mind.

VL DEALEXANDER

Intermittent Fasting

TIPS, EATING PATTERN, AND MEALS

My 10 Year Journey of How Intermittent Fasting Changed My Life Making Me Feel Lighter, Healthier, and Full of Energy

by VL DeAlexander

INTERMITTENT FASTING

CONTENTS

INTRODUCTION   1

CHAPTER 1: Year 1: Not Healthy, Nor Ill ... Just   5
Average

CHAPTER 2: Year 1: Intermittent Fasting, Why Not?   9

What is Intermittent fasting?

CHAPTER 3: Year 1: I tried Everything and Here's   15
What I Came Up With

Conclusion

CHAPTER 4: Benefits of Intermittent Fasting   21

Conclusion

CHAPTER 5: Year 2: The Obstacles: Pain and   27
Struggle

Mistake #1: Not Keeping the Time

Mistake #2: Lack of Hydration

Mistake #3: No Accountability

Mistake #4: Drinking My Coffee with Cream and Sugar

Mistake #5: Eating Too Much of the Wrong Kinds of Foods

Mistake #6: Doing Too Much Activity While Fasting

My Recommendations for You

Conclusion

CHAPTER 6: Year 3: Cooking My Own Meals   35

How Cooking at Home Helped Me

What Types of Things Did I Cook?

What Was My Budged for the Food?

My Recommendations for You on This Adventure

Why Your Diet is Important

Conclusion

CHAPTER 7: Diet Plans for Intermittent Fasting   42

1. The 8-6 Meal Plan

2. The 12-6 Meal Plan

3. The 2-Day Plan

4. The 5-2 Plan

5. Every-Other-Day Plan

The Warrior Diet

Conclusion

CHAPTER 8: Years 5-6: Workout and Intermittent Fasting   57

Exercising While Fasting

The Solution to Dealing with the Challenges

My Example

How It Can Help You Lose Weight

Conclusion

CHAPTER 9: Years 7-10: Benefits I Am Seeing in My Body   64

What All This Means for You

Conclusion

CHAPTER 10: The Man I Am Today (10 Years Later)   72

CHAPTER 11: Powerful Tips to Make You Start Now   76

How Long Do You Want to Fast?

What Are Some of the Side Effects That I Might Encounter?

What Are Some of the Things to Keep in Mind During a Fast?

Who Shouldn't Fast?

How to Begin Now

Conclusion

CONCLUSION OF CHAPTERS   87

INTRODUCTION

Every man and woman desire to look hot and fit. They want to be attractive and be able to date whoever they like. Not every person can achieve this feat, however. Too many people are struggling with their weight. They're not eating right, and are putting on the fat and calories. Too many people have just let it go and have not taken care of themselves. I realize that I fell into this trap too many times ten years ago when I was but 28-years old, young and single without a wife to take care of. I was a graduate of a liberal arts college with a degree in communications and was drifting through life. Because I didn't have a girlfriend, I wanted to do something more. And later….I found intermittent fasting.

This book is about how I, Victor Lorenzo DeAlexander, became fit with a hot body by doing intermittent fasting and exercise. I am going to introduce each part of my story and include anecdotes and stories that I hope will inspire you to begin a chapter of fasting and exercise. I told you every person wants to look hot and fit, but they don't know how to get there. I think that there is definitely a way to achieve this, but you can't just sit there on your ass and do nothing about it; you have to take action. You have to have a plan. Too much of a person's life is spent in contemplation and complacency and not enough action. People are guilty of not following through with their words, and there are inconsistencies between what they say and what they do.

But you don't want to be that person, I think. You want to be a person of integrity, a person who is true to yourself and wants to accomplish your goals because you are worth it. I believe that every person should be able to reach their objectives if they set realistic, concrete, and achievable goals. That is the only way that they can do it, and I believe that you can also achieve your dreams.

I'm telling my story because it worked. Intermittent fasting changed my life. It made me realize what was important in my life, saved me a boatload of money, and made me feel and look healthier. I also got a hot bod that all the ladies were admiring, and, as a result, I became more confident and happy about my life. It helped me so much, and I believe that you can also do it. I think that you are a person with a purpose. Too many people go through life without a goal, but I believe that you can do it as well. You can get a sexy body because you have a dream to do so. That dream is real and tangible, but you have to believe that it is also something you can reach for and attain. Nothing is impossible. You must understand that all things are possible with a mindset that is positive and growth-oriented.

In this book, I have organized my ideas based on the story that I want to narrate. I show what caused me to go on this journey with intermittent fasting, what worked and what didn't, how I changed my diet and eating patterns, what I did to improve my workout routines, the benefits I have encountered, and the recommendations and tips that I think will help you to build the body of your dreams.

Each chapter is organized with an introduction, life story and lesson, and conclusion, so that you can follow each tip carefully and effectively. I have made this book one that you can reflect on, and it is conversational in nature so that you can pretend that you are in a meeting with me. Imagine we are talking together over a beer or coffee about ways that you can achieve this dream that you have had maybe since you were a boy or girl or teenager. I want you to feel empowered to reach the goal that you've had. It is possible for you to do it. I believe in you. Trust me on this and come with me on this journey. Together, we can achieve what you want. I am offering this book as a means for you to be supported and guided on this journey, based on my own experiences. It will be rough at some points. It was difficult for me, too. I suffered from some severe bouts, but it was all worth it. Like the adage says, "no pain, no gain." You have to take it as it comes. The battle can be fierce and cruel at times, but it is something worth fighting for. There are difficult and great things about this intermittent fasting that I want to share with you, but I also want to show you how to do it and get the results desired.

CHAPTER 1

(YEAR 1)

NOT HEALTHY, NOR ILL … JUST AVERAGE

In this chapter, I will introduce how I was at the beginning of my journey to better health. I will explain my story in the beginning as an average man looking to improve my health after many essential circumstances.

In the beginning, I, Victor, was just an average guy. There was no ambition in my life. I didn't have a goal that I was going for. Instead, I was just coasting through life, trying to figure out what I wanted to do. Having gone to college, I got my degree in communications. It was a kind of default major that people take just because they want to get a degree. After I graduated, I didn't have a lot of money. I had $30,000 in school debt I had to pay back to my university. When I left school, I could not get a job in my field. I wanted to be a radio host on a radio station in my town. I had, in my mind, an idea to remain in my hometown for the rest of my life. I didn't want to move out on my own, or get my own place. Because I was making less than $20,000 a year working at Starbucks and tutoring on the side, I wasn't able to become financially well-off.

As for my health, I was in pretty good shape. I ate ok. Sometimes, I went out and got drunk and would go clubbing with my friends. I ate at McDonald's frequently, so I gained some weight. Occasionally, I would smoke cigarettes with friends outside. I also went to the Hookah bar sometimes to socialize. The kind of exercise I got was just enough to get by. I went to the gym once or twice a week. I was not maintaining a healthy weight, and had put on a few pounds by snacking every night after dinner.

Although I did some unhealthy things, I could say that I was in average health and didn't have too much going for me. There wasn't too much to comment about it. As I said, I was coasting through my life with no ambition. No desire to get married or settle down. All I wanted to do was stay in my parents' basement and use my hard-earned money from Starbucks to pay my bills and student loans. In that time, I was not happy. I felt trapped by my situation. I wanted to get out of it. I was unsure about how I could proceed. Wasn't there something else I could try for in my life? Why did I always have to eat away my feelings and indulge in little things that were unhealthy? I just thought to myself; it doesn't matter. I'll be this way for a little while, and, eventually, I'll settle down and get married. Right now, I can settle for going out, getting drunk sometimes, going to a club, and working at Starbucks. Later, I can think about going back to school and getting my shit together.

On the surface, you might say I was doing all right. I was just like any average American young man. I didn't have a goal or purpose in life, and indulged in pleasures. That was the way it was with many twenty-somethings out there. Many young people these days are lost. They don't know where to go with their lives. They graduate with so much debt and then can't find a job that will help them repay those loans. I was one of those people. I was among the many people who are struggling to find their way amid this broken system in America. The education system is broken. The job market is broken, and I was one of the people who had to suffer from it.

It was one day when I was 28 that I thought to myself, "What am I doing with my life?" "Why am I stuck in this shithole?" "Why can't I try to get out?" And I realized that I was quite complacent in dealing with the underlying issue of what to do with my life. I was procrastinating. When I lost my mother to breast cancer, I received a wake-up call. I realized that life was painfully short and that I had to do something to live a healthier and more productive life. I had to take inventory of my life and see how I was doing with my health so that I could get a new action plan.

Realizing that life was short and that I had to do something to prolong my life in a good way that does not extend my adolescence, I started looking for a way to do that. I decided to stop procrastinating. I looked up ways to be healthy and read some books about healthy eating and living. I knew I needed an action plan and soon, I would discover what I wanted to do: intermittent fasting.

To conclude, I was able to realize what was important to me. What was important to me was finding a solution to my problem of unhealthy habits. I came up with the answer - to follow a regimen of intermittent fasting that would give me the chance to maintain a healthy weight and to be able to do a lot of great things in my life. Everything is possible, I know that, and I looked forward to seeing what was going to happen.

CHAPTER 2

(YEAR 1)

INTERMITTENT FASTING, WHY NOT?

In this chapter, I will explain how I came up with my decision to give intermittent fasting a try. The media provided me with a source of inspiration, and I was eager to begin this journey into better health, looking good, and feeling great. Here is the story of what happened.

One day, I was on my Netflix binge. Since it was my day off from Starbucks, I was on my computer in my parents' basement, and I had already enjoyed sleeping-in after a long weekend. I then went on YouTube and binged more on videos and things. I did an extensive search of different healthy eating options and ways to live a better life. Suddenly, there was a video that played, and it was Hugh Jackman in X-Men as Wolverine. I saw his amazing body and thought I really wanted to be that guy. He was so ripped and was also quite attractive. Later, I found out how Hugh Jackman was able to get this lean, ripped Wolverine body through a diet from intermittent fasting. Jackman is one of my favorite actors and heroes. I look up to the man. He has been one of my icons. He talked about all the advantages of doing intermittent fasting and how it can benefit your health. And then I thought, "That's it!" "Sweet!" I knew, at that point, that I wanted to do intermittent fasting. I tried to engage in a habit that my hero did, and wanted to be just like him.

That's when I decided that I wanted to do something just for myself to build up my confidence in my body. I knew I had flab and didn't have muscle mass. I tried to look like Wolverine and get big abs and a sexy body that every woman would want. I decided that I really wanted to get healthier and do what Hugh Jackman does. He eats for 8 hours and then fasts for 16 hours. In the YouTube video I watched, he said that most of what a person looks like comes from their diet and what they eat, so I realized that to get buff and fit, I needed to look at my diet and see what I could do to get the physique that I wanted.

To be honest, this was the most ambitious thing that I could try to do. Getting into shape was an essential part of the process because I wanted to take action. I tried to get the body of a sexy dude. I knew that I had to set this goal for myself. It was so important to me. Nothing else had worked for me. I didn't have an action plan for my life. I was still coasting through life, switching my part-time job every year or two but, with this goal, I knew I had something I didn't have before. I was ready for it; I was going to try this intermittent fasting thing.

From the moment of deciding how to do intermittent fasting, I went online and found the different ways people did it and looked at their stories. I became inspired and thought to myself "Why not?" I want to do the same thing. It seems like a great way to get fit and a way to lose the unhealthy lifestyle that I was living in. I then went online and found how you could do this intermittent fasting plan and I started to set some goals for myself, how I wanted to see myself in one month, two months, or in one year. I started charting my feelings and thoughts. It was a fantastic moment for me, and I knew that I could do anything. Perhaps, I would be able to find meaning for my life, because I knew just how important it was to take care of your body.

What is Intermittent Fasting?

In short, it is a way to get your body in shape by not eating for some time. You have an abstemious appetite and can eat adequately for a given time, and then you stop eating and do exercise, and then you go to sleep, wake up, rinse and repeat. You may have reservations about what fasting can do for you because, perhaps, you have heard how hard it is and how you'll get headaches, feel nauseous and not good at times. Well, that's probably going to be the beginning for you. It always sucks in the beginning, but once you get started and get into a routine, it will feel like riding a bike, and you will see and feel the result.

Intermittent fasting has been used by people throughout the world, including Gandhi, Jesus, and other amazing people. You may think it is for the religious and ascetics, but it's not. Anyone can fast. It doesn't always have to have a spiritual component, although, if you're into God, it will help you get close to that transcendent being and will bring you more in-tune with your thoughts and spiritual world. Fasting enables you to be in tune with your spirit and how it works, because, once you stop consuming food, your body is fed not through the physical sensations, but through the elements of the spirit. Your mind is able to focus on the experiences that impact your soul. Intermittent fasting is surprisingly simple and is used by many people around the world. As soon as you have started the routine, you will find that it is so natural that you will think, "How did I not do this before?" It became something that I wanted to do.

Not eating may sound like it's no big deal. After all, living life for saying "no" to the excesses of life seems out of place for this world. Most people love to boast about which restaurant they went to by posting on Instagram, Facebook etc., and showing pictures of their food. But what if there is a simpler way to do it? That's why I decided to do something simpler and more fruitful that could contribute to a lifestyle change. My life needed to be transformed, so I chose the path of least resistance and did something I would say is "minimalistic," in greatly simplifying my life. I have to say, it has made the most significant difference in my life. I am no longer the same man.

In what follows, I am going to show you how this life of intermittent fasting has transformed my life, how it has made me into the man I am today, and how it has led me from being a chubby, no-abs man to a fit and healthy man with a six-pack, who is happy and free. The thing that you have to realize is that you have to set a goal for yourself. You have to set the standard high. No more mediocrity; no more settling for less. You have to own the man or woman that you want to become. You have to hold within your hands the person that you aim to be. You cannot live your life without a goal or objective to go after. Too many people are drifting through their lives, trying to figure out where they should go.

I'm telling you, don't be that person. You have to pursue your passion and do it with zeal. I have learned from this new experience of intermittent fasting that I wanted to achieve an ideal body, diet, and lifestyle. The way to do that was to take the necessary steps and measures. I just had to have a dream and then go after it with all my might. So, what are you waiting for? Let's go on this journey. It is a long journey through my life, but it is a fantastic reflection of how self-discipline, goal-setting, and a bit of hard work and determination have paid off and led me to be a successful man today.

CHAPTER 3

(YEAR 1)

I TRIED EVERYTHING AND HERE'S WHAT I CAME UP WITH

This chapter covers my experience in year 1 when I tried everything to get my weight and diet in order, but nothing was working. I finally tried intermittent fasting and it changed my life. It took some time, but then I sorted it out and decided I would give it a try and that it would change my eating habits. In this chapter, I am going to show you what I did, and then tell you what I'd recommend that you do.

As I was looking for weight management and increasing muscle, I realized I would have to work super hard to get the results I wanted. I tried all the diet plans, including all carb diet, diets filled with protein, and other ones. They always made me feel bloated and not very good. I also tried to take protein powder while I was working out. That didn't work out too well. I was very unhappy with my body type and wanted to seek some help for my situation. I had no idea what to do. The more I worked out, the more weight I was losing because my metabolism was working on overdrive and there was no slowing it down. Also, I tried to eat every 2 hours and then gorged myself with huge meals during lunch to try to get myself to gain weight. I ended up stuffing my face all day, and I felt miserable, had stomach aches, and just felt like crap overall.

My workout routines were not healthy as well. I was running on the treadmill for 2 hours a day and doing cardio like crazy. I was swimming laps four times a week for 1 hour a day. I was also deadlifting four times a week and trying my best to build up muscle while packing my stomach with food. I even took snacks with me to the gym to eat right away once my workout routine had finished. I was racing against time to get myself into shape. It was so freaking difficult. I could never keep up my metabolism with my workouts. It was impossible to do it. I was literally consuming 4,000 calories a day and burning almost all of it because I was exercising so much. And it felt pointless. I was not completing my goals but, then again, I didn't really have any reachable goals. Everything was just put together in a not-so-formal way. I didn't really know what I was doing in this process of trying to buff up. I was not convinced that I could do it.

Looking back at it, I was not doing well. I was trying to manage everything in my own strength and power. I had a poor body image, struggled with who I looked like, and didn't even want to look at myself in the mirror, yet, I aspired to have the body of Arnold Schwarzenegger, or other famous actors with amazing bodies. Knowing that I wanted to get this body and workout, all the same, I wanted to have some options with what I could do, and how I could achieve my goal of that great body that every woman wants to see on a guy.

It was at this point that I decided I had no other option. I needed to do something that would help me to get on track. Intermittent fasting was the option that I chose based on research and looking up different information about how to do it, and I was immediately struck at how easy it was to begin a wellness routine with this method and habit. It just requires you to abstain from food for a period of time. Intermittent fasting allows yourself to take in calories and protein for some time, and work out with the given energy you have. You are then able to see the results of your efforts.

Reflecting on this experience, I realize that millions of people are in this situation. Maybe you are too. You don't know what to do with what you've got. You are unsure how to proceed with your workout routine and diet, so you pack on the protein with shakes, powders and pills. You may also be a person who is working out like crazy and wants to try to add more weight by eating so much to try to increase your metabolic rate. Well, I'm here to tell you, that will not work. It may for a short period, but, after a while, you will either lose that weight which will be burnt off, or you will gain some fat in the process, mainly if you overeat fat or calories. Take heart though, you can achieve your dreams and goals. You should not give up on trying to find the solution. You should not try to do too much or overeat. It is vital that you designate a place for rest and do nothing. Too much workout or food is not going to solve the problems for you. You will need to find ways of relaxing and give yourself breaks from time to time. Additionally, you will have to find a way to use your creativity to live a productive life that is filled with activity and joy. Find an outlet that will help you, whether that is painting, writing, watching films, hanging out with friends, or joining a club.

There is a better way to find the solution to your weight problem, and it is so simple. I tried it, and it worked. Intermittent fasting is going to change your life. Within this method, you will realize that you can seamlessly integrate it into your busy life, and it won't be too difficult. You will be able to accomplish great things by eating only one or two meals a day. You will realize that you can do everything you set your mind to! Nothing is impossible.

When you feel like eating that pizza or burger, go right ahead, because you will be fasting from calories for one or two meals a day. Enjoy! You can find that this routine is going to change and shape the way you eat and work out. No more counting the calories or fat content. You can enjoy a life of freedom and high energy that will make every feat possible.

Conclusion

From what I've told you, I want you to think about giving intermittent fasting a try. You won't be the same person again. You will see the world through a new lens, like never before. If you follow my advice, you will find yourself able to achieve what seemed impossible before. If you do what I tell you to do, you will be able to lose those pounds that you put on because you didn't eat right. Also, you will be able to get that hot body that you always wanted, and you will be super fit because you can follow a workout routine that will help you to build muscle mass.

I'm Victor, your guide on this journey. I've been there, done that. You can trust me because I have seen and done it all. Throughout my 10-year voyage, I saw a lot of development in my own body and workout routine, and I believe that you will also see amazing results. I want to be here to support you through your time. I tried it all and then came to this point where I could do nothing else. Allow me to guide you through this thing. We can do it all together. Don't be afraid or anxious. This journey is meant to be done with someone else. Let me and a friend or buddy help you to achieve your goal. All things will happen at the right time. I'll cheer you on the whole way.

CHAPTER 4

BENEFITS OF INTERMITTENT FASTING

Now that you have chosen to give intermittent fasting a try, I want to educate you about the benefits of intermittent fasting that have been proven by research. In this chapter, I will highlight the types of things that you can get out of pursuing this life of wellness. Here are some things to bear in mind as you are feeling more motivated to do this thing.

You may be wondering, why not eat whenever I want? Why shouldn't I just eat as much as I want of healthy food sources? In my opinion, if you give your whole system a break from food and give your stomach some rest time, you will see a wide range of benefits that I want you to see for yourself:

• Lowers the risk of cancer. One study has proven that when you modify the frequency and timing of eating, you can influence the use of insulin and decrease the risk for breast cancer in women.

• Helps you have a healthy heart. Intermittent fasting can lower your risk of heart disease because your triglycerides and blood pressure are reduced and it also gives you healthy cholesterol. I went to the cardiologist for a test last year, and I was able to find out that my heart was healthy, as if it were 25! That means that this intermittent fasting is doing something for me.

• Helps you to lose weight quickly. Intermittent fasting is going to help you to lose weight faster as you can lessen leptin resistance, which causes your body to store fat for energy instead of burning it (William Cole). While I didn't have a problem directly with this, I was able to successfully manage my weight over time after doing intermittent fasting as I've mentioned above.

• Allows you to stop craving so much food during the day. When you do intermittent fasting, you will stop craving food when you're hungry. I'll be honest about this one. I used to snack all the time and gained some fat on my belly as a result. I was not a happy camper. Once I started intermittent fasting, I realized that I could go for stretches of time without snacking. It was amazing!

• Helps to improve your lungs. Another study has shown that intermittent fasting can decrease symptoms of asthma, as well as stress (William Cole). For this one, I was able to improve my lungs over time. I had my full body scan, and the doctor said my lungs were super healthy. I was delighted to hear that point.

Intermittent fasting helps you with your overall energy levels. When you store energy from your food, you're able to release it when you're active again. Usually, this will entail working out during the period when you eat, and then resting during fasting periods. You will notice a tangible difference in your energy level and feel more hyper and energetic as a result of these fasts.

You will feel happier and more productive. I felt the difference and was sincerely happy when I first started this type of fasting. It made me feel like I was "on top of the world" and I could do anything I wanted. There is a seriously empowering feeling that you experience whenever you are doing this intermittent fasting routine.

You will struggle less with depression and anxiety. When you eat healthily and do the right kind of exercise, you will find that you can get less anxious or depressed. A lot of what we eat determines what our moods will be like, so the best thing is to stick to a plan that will strengthen our immune system and help us to feel better. I was able to enjoy my food and have a period of no eating. It helped me to feel secure and it stabled my moods because the fat was being stored in my body over time. It was great.

These are some of the benefits I have been able to find out while researching and pondering. There are a host of others that I was able to discover, but I wanted to inform you about what I was able to find. Intermittent fasting will be a type of program you want to be on, not just for the short-term, but for the long-term, as well. It is going to help you achieve long-term health benefits because you're willing to submit to a disciplined program that will work wonders for your lungs, gut, and heart. I'm telling you it is worth it!

I know I had some difficulties motivating myself to do this. I didn't want to have to skip a meal a day and go for periods where I would be hungry. Believe me, it can feel like a huge sacrifice that you're making every time you do this but, after I read about the benefits, I felt more motivated to keep going with it. Research has extensively proven the effectiveness of intermittent fasting, and that's where I knew that I was doing the right thing. If many scientists were proving how great it was, then I knew that it was going to be something that would work wonders in my life.

So, what are you waiting for? Don't you believe in the power of science and research? They support the decisions I make in my life. You also have to follow what research is saying because, often, these studies are proving the point that you should do something to improve your overall health, and the majority of studies have shown the positive aspects of intermittent fasting. No wonder so many people are getting into it today. They see how intermittent fasting helps them get into shape, benefits their immune system, and gives them a sense of purpose and meaning to their lives. People know that this type of fasting is going to help them get their health on the right track. No more worrying about what goes into their stomach or uselessly counting of all the sugar and fats that a person is taking in. That's nonsense. Don't waste your time on the things that are not effective. Do things that are proven to work. Intermittent fasting is going to help you do just that.

Conclusion

To conclude, as I was thinking about intermittent fasting, I realized that science was proving just how great it was. I am a believer in the progress of humanity and that, through scientific achievements, we can make the world a better place. Having examined the research that has been conducted on this topic, I knew that I wanted to educate people on how wonderful intermittent fasting could be. I hope that you will see how you can also benefit from it.

CHAPTER 5

(YEAR 2)

THE OBSTACLES: PAIN AND STRUGGLE

In this chapter, I am going to be frank and candid about the struggles and pain that went into intermittent fasting during my second year. I will share my insights on how I handled these situations and then I will go into tips for coping with the challenges that you will inevitably face. I am also going to offer you some solutions.

When I first started fasting, it was a hard time for me. I felt anxious the first few days I was trying to fast because I was scared of not eating at my regular times. I was also afraid of losing muscle mass because I was not eating. I thought I would lose more weight than gain any, so I was quite skeptical about it. Also, I felt ashamed that I was trying this method because I thought my parents would not approve and that they would make fun of me for trying to do this fasting. I also thought that people would not understand and think I was starving myself. I would get criticism from everyone I met because they would say to me, "Victor, you're so skinny. You shouldn't be starving yourself. You have to feed yourself with something. Eat a burger from Burger King. Do something to up your fat and calories." That would make me feel ashamed and embarrassed.

In the past, I had told my friends and family that I wanted to become a pescatarian or a vegan. Within a few weeks, I quit doing it, because they said to me I need to eat more meat and carbs. I listened to them; therefore, I felt cautious about giving people information that I was going to start fasting.

As for my physique, I had a lot of fat on my body. Although I was lean, I struggled with strength training. I was overeating and cultivating some seriously bad habits. Unfortunately, those bad habits caused me a lot of heartaches as I was starting the plan. I began the program with many mistakes that I want to share with you. They were difficult, and I learned from them, but they caused me a great deal of pain.

Mistake #1: Not Keeping the Time

The first mistake I made in doing this plan was not watching the clock. Basically, I would eat whenever I felt hungry. In the beginning, I didn't have set meal times and would just eat anytime but, as I started the intermittent fasting, I realized that I had to have set meal times that I could sit down and have my meal. I realized that I had to program myself so that I could do that, but I was so lazy and only wanted to feel satisfied. As a result, I got off to a rough start and didn't lose any weight during my second year.

Mistake #2: Lack of Hydration

The second mistake I made was not being hydrated through the day. As a result, I got these intense headaches that were horrible. I even had to go into hospital for not hydrating my body correctly. It hurt like crap. I was so miserable. At that hospital visit, I thought I was going to die, both of thirst and hunger. The doctor had to plug up an IV to me to keep me hydrated. Never again.

Mistake #3: No Accountability

The third mistake I made was not having someone to keep me accountable. Every person needs a trusted friend to help them to make it through. No accountability = no progress. I felt that I needed to have someone to check in with me throughout this process, but I was stubborn and thought, "Oh, ok, I'm fine. I'll just deal with it all on my own."

Mistake #4: Drinking My Coffee with Cream and Sugar

For a while, I thought I could deal with the problem of hunger by drinking more coffee, and that would help me make it through; then I started cheating on my calories. I started adding milk or cream and sugar to my coffee to make it just like a meal and, when I did that, I inadvertently stopped my fast. This was something that I shouldn't have done, but I was doing it, all the same. Now I realize it was dishonest and I shouldn't have done it. If you're drinking coffee, drink it straight black with no added ingredients.

Mistake #5: Eating Too Much of the Wrong Kinds of Food

I started out with this chapter talking about how I ate a lot of junk food. I would eat pizza, burgers, chips, among other kinds of junk food, all because they would fill me up and I would feel satisfied in the end. When I became 30-years old, I realized I had to get better at my eating habits. I needed to eat foods that not only were going to satisfy me and fill my stomach, but also benefit my health. I had to change from filling up on so many high-calorie foods, so I had to make some changes to my diet.

Mistake #6: Doing Too Much Activity While Fasting

When I started with intermittent fasting, I did too much heavy lifting and exercised in my fasting period, and I began to lose some muscle from all that training. I checked my weight after a few times of fasting and exercise, and I would lose 3-5 pounds at a time. Because I am lean, I could lose weight super quick, so keeping on weight was quite the challenge for me. Having too much workout and activity caused me to lose weight and muscle, which was not helpful for me, as I wanted to get a healthier body type and a fit physique like the Wolverine.

During the period of the first two years, I was struggling to get into a routine of fasting. I tried different things, got too ambitious, wanted to find some ways of coping with hunger pain and other things, and ended up having some unfortunate experiences. I had to learn a lot about how to do the intermittent fasting based on the different available plans. I wanted to quit. I'm not going to lie. It sucked sometimes. I was struggling to have a reason to keep going, and I also ended up having some depression and mental health issues, as well. I realized that it was hard for me and I needed someone to support me through this time.

My Recommendations for You

What I recommend you do is not making the same mistakes that I made. First of all, don't go in without planning how you're going to do your fast, or how long you will do it for. Plan for failure. You have to go in with a plan, knowing exactly how you're going to execute it. Secondly, you will need to drink a lot of water during your fast. Because your body is burning calories while you're fasting, you will need to replenish its supply of water. Don't make the mistake of having to go into hospital like me and have an IV connected to you. It's just not worth it. Thirdly, drink your coffee black. Don't add anything to it. Don't try to cheat your way to fasting. It's not honest, and it's lying to yourself and others. You have to be a person of integrity, and the only way that you'll get ahead with this is by following the guidelines of fasting. Fourthly, find someone you know who you can tell about your plan to fast. Allow that trusted friend to be your accountability partner. Talk to that person and tell them when you're fasting, so that they can be a supportive person. Fifthly, you should talk to your doctor about your plan. Let them know that you're planning on doing intermittent fasting. It's crucial that they understand what you're going to do so they can make health recommendations that you should listen to. Next, you have to eat the right kinds of foods. In the sixth chapter, I will go into what types of foods you definitely should eat. You don't want to fall into the trap of eating the wrong kinds of foods because that will not help you achieve your weight-management goals. Finally, exercise in a reasonable frame of time with good intensity. You want to do your best, but don't overdo it, because that will be counterproductive and will not enable you to finish what you start. Fit in a workout plan that will help you eat during a designated period. Also, you should find a time to rest your body from all the working out that you might be doing. It's vital that your body finds times to rest from all the energy that it is exerting.

Conclusion

As you can see, there are certain things that you should avoid in your intermittent fasting plan. You don't want to be without a plan at all. You have to be specific with your goals and stick to your project. Don't deviate from what you have written down as your plan. You also have to be careful to watch out for all the health concerns that there might be. Without the proper consultation with a physician, you might be in for trouble, so talk to your doctor before you start a plan. Finally, maintain a healthy balance with exercise, diet, and rest, and you will be on your way to a successful routine that could change your life.

CHAPTER 6

(YEAR 3)

COOKING MY OWN MEALS

This chapter discusses one strategy that I used to become healthier - cooking my own meals. I will give you some of the tips and strategies that I used to make this part of my wellness routine work.

When I first started thinking about how I would do this intermittent fasting thing, I realized that I wanted to make myself healthier, so I stopped going to McDonald's and eating fried foods all the time. I then discovered that I actually liked to cook. I guess I only needed to give it some time; enough time for me to make a delicious recipe or something that I would like that's also super healthy. In the following paragraphs, I will explain how cooking my own meals transformed my way of thinking and led me to a new chapter in my life.

First, once I got the diabetes diagnosis, I knew that I needed to take inventory over my fat and sugar intake. It was getting way out of control. I was eating too many fried foods and drinking fizzy drinks. It was getting out of hand. I was also spending too much on food every month. There was just too much. Too much on the portion sizes. Too much on the cost. I lived for excess. I finally had an epiphany in which I realized I needed to eat more healthily or else I would become obese; therefore, I decided to cook my own meals — the best decision I could make.

As a single man living alone, I wanted to figure out how to cook the best and most delicious meals that I could make. I watched Food Network and Martha Stewart Living for more information. Don't laugh at me. Those are good shows, even for men looking to up their game in the kitchen. Instead of spending a lot of money on drinks and going out with friends, I ended up spending the money on organic food with fruits and vegetables from different stores, such as Greenlife. It was the best investment for me, and I ended up saving around $200 each month on all that food. It was great. Furthermore, that money could go back into the debt payments that I needed to make every month. It worked out well with my finances.

How Cooking at Home Helped Me

Cooking at home was a great thing because I didn't look to be going out all the time to eat any longer. I could stay in and make amazing fancy meals for one. I could also focus on what was the most important thing for me - enjoying life and being a "live-to-eat" person, rather than an "eat-to-leave" type. I also started to slow down as I ate my meals. I truly enjoyed the opportunity to indulge in every bite of my Fettuccine Alfredo, courtesy of Giada De Laurentiis. It was amazing to discover all the best recipes on the Food Network and apply them to my kitchen and, at the age of 30, I started to invest in the cookware that would make me enjoy working in my kitchen. It was fantastic. Cooking at home was also the answer to my weight-management plan. I was able to eat well and not spend too much money. I had to come up with ways to make things better for myself, so I resorted to cooking my meals, and it made a huge difference.

What Types of Things Did I Cook?

As I got more creative with cooking, I realized that there is not much you have to do to get the results that you want. All you have to do is use the same essential ingredients and then you can do almost anything with those ingredients. I started with making eggs, bacon, and biscuits, which would give me a high carb and protein diet. I realized that I needed to cook more of protein and carbs because I had low muscle mass and was a very skinny person. I had very little in the way of muscles. Because I had eaten just any way I wanted before, I was struggling to get rid of my fat that was on my belly. I also wanted to gain more weight, but also increase muscle mass. I started cooking meals such as pasta carbonara that had cheese, egg, and bacon. This helped me to develop a repertoire of healthy and filling meals, but it wasn't just the carbohydrates that I added to my diet. I also made salads - green salads. I developed a desire to make my balsamic vinaigrette and added feta cheese, mushrooms, tomatoes, and green peppers to make a delicious meal. I then added a few slices of toast with avocado spread to the mix. It was amazing. I made so many simple meals that I was able to enjoy daily, and I didn't feel the temptation to go out and splurge on that meal at a restaurant. Going out can easily cost a fortune from $20 - 25 in a regular restaurant, and I didn't want to break the bank anymore. It was too much for me.

What Was My Budget for the Food?

Before starting this routine of cooking my meals, I was easily blowing over $500 on food and drink. Every night I was going to a restaurant with friends or having a glass of wine with my meals. I was doing so much work that I had no desire to go home and prepare my lunch because I was so exhausted from the job. Many times I would order delivery at $30 a pop for pizza and wine or beer. I was entirely frivolous with my expenses and did not watch what I was spending and ended up with very little money at the end of the month. Unfortunately, I was careless. After starting this new routine, I noticed I was a lot more careful with my expenses and looked at my wallet and made the right decisions, especially when it came to grocery shopping. I have no regrets. It was a great thing to do, and I am thankful it all worked out the way it did.

My Recommendations for You on this Adventure

As I consider what is essential, I believe that making your own meals at home is very productive and also healthy. If you go to a restaurant, you never know how many hands have been touching that burger or fry that you order. Also, it is quite uncomfortable to be in a restaurant eating all the time, where there are a lot of germs, not to mention the fact that so many additives are put on the food that makes it quite unhealthy. This is why I am all for the idea of finding ways to prepare food at home. It's not hard.

The main thing you need to do is to master the basics of cooking at home. You have to find a few ingredients and make the same meal over and over with those ingredients. Go online and search for ways you can spice it up by adding ingredients or using a different recipe. Consult Food Network or Martha Stewart. You can always find some creative ways to spice up that PB&J or grilled cheese. There are so many recipes out there you can try. All you have to do is go online, and you will find the solutions there. Find the best ingredients you can. You can order your food online, or go to the store and pick everything out on your own. It is essential to find the right ingredients that will be healthy with no additives and no MSGs. This is crucial to giving you a healthy diet.

Why Your Diet is Important

In addition to the tips about cooking at home, you should know just how important it is to keep your diet under control. If you want to buff up or develop a better body, you will have to watch what you eat. You should eat lots of protein, carbs, fruit and vegetables. A balanced diet is so vital to giving you the result that you desire. The only way you're going to get fit is by focusing mostly on your diet because that will influence how you get more muscle mass. I realized I wasn't eating right and that was why, no matter how much I went to the gym, I was still not getting the results that I wanted in my muscles; therefore, I recommend focusing on how you can make your diet the best that it can be.

Conclusion

My conclusion is that diet and making your meals at home will give you a wellness routine like no other. You have to learn to slow down. This world is too fast-paced. We go through the drive-thru at McDonald's when we feel like it. Too much of the food we consume is fast food and full of MSGs and additives that are quite toxic and can cause sickness or worse. I had a crisis of discovering I had diabetes that made me watch what I ate and helped me to take control of the fat and other things I consumed. Don't wait until it's too late to find a solution to this problem. Act now. Your health is so important. Take good care of yourself.

CHAPTER 7

DIET PLANS FOR INTERMITTENT FASTING

In this chapter, I will talk in detail about how I started to develop the diet plans that would help me as I did my intermittent fasting. I will talk about my story, and then I will offer you some recommendations for what you can do to get the most out of your diet plan.

During my third year, I had started developing my meals at home. This was the first time that I had gotten my own place, so I was super excited. Armed with the knowledge that I had about intermittent fasting, I wanted to cook some super simple meals at home.

I'm now going to talk about some diet plans that worked for me and helped me to manage my weight and energy levels all the time. I will start out with the program that helped me the most in the beginning. I did some research on this matter, so I could get it right. I will show you what I did at each step of the process, so you can get an idea of what you can do for your diet plan.

When you start your intermittent fasting journey, you will probably see that you feel fuller for a more extended period, and that you will be able to eat more naturally. In the following plans, I will show you what I did for each part of it, and how I fitted in the meal times around my fasting schedule.

1.   The 8-6 Meal Plan

Here is an example of what I did for a while at the beginning of my fasting. I would eat between the hours of 8am and 6pm. I was able to find the right balance with fasting and eating and get a taste of what it was like to fast. It was still a 14-hour fast, and it was instrumental in helping me to improve my metabolism. Let me show you what I ate during that time.

Breakfast: Avocado   smoothie   with blueberries at 8am

In the morning, I would begin my day with a protein-packed smoothie that was easier to digest having fasted the night before. Often, I would get sick when eating breakfast in the morning because I would feel woozy and not very good. In the beginning, I started by binging on pancakes, biscuits, bacon and eggs. I realized that this was not healthy and that I was killing my weight plan goals, so I soon resorted to smoothies in the morning, which helped me to get going before I would have lunch at noon. The ingredients of my smoothie would include protein powder, avocado, kale, chia seeds, blueberries, and coconut milk. Basically, I would grab all of these ingredients, put them in the blender, and go to town with it. It felt great, and I soon realized that I was eating healthier and having a higher level of energy. It did wonders for my health.

Lunch: Veggie burgers at 12:30pm

During the week, I went to Greenlife grocery and would get veggie burgers, which are packed with energy. They are simple, but effective to cook at home. In addition to the veggie burger, I would put leafy lettuce on top of them, garlic powder, and cumin to top it off. It was always delicious and easy to prepare. I would cook them on the stove top at home and put them on a bun. It was a great way to cook and have a good meal at home.

Snack: Cinnamon rolls at 3pm

I didn't have to skimp on sugar intake during this time, so I would give myself a meal around 3pm, and it was terrific. I was able to provide myself with some sugar and fat right before dinner. Cinnamon rolls are quite delicious and also easy to prepare. You just have to give yourself the time to do it during the day.

Dinner: Tuna and veggies at 6pm

Fish can be a great way to get your omega-3 fats in your diet. I love to eat tuna salad from time to time. You can also make this into a sandwich, which is particularly delicious. For example, you can go to the bakery and get a baguette slice or something and then add it to this mix. Then, you can stir fry some vegetables. Add yogurt or a cookie for dessert, and you have a great meal at the end of your day, which is high in nutrients.

This plan worked for me for a couple of years. I was struggling to find a way to eat at designated times, so, when I tried this plan, I was able to schedule my eating between this window, and it helped me to achieve even better results. This plan can be used for beginners, who are just starting with their fasting routines. As I went along, I wanted to challenge myself to fast for more extended periods, and it was at that point that I was able to make even more progress with my wellness plan. As I went with the 8-6 program, I started to notice how my appetite would get more abstemious, and I no longer felt too hungry or had a stomach rumbling throughout my day.

2. The 12-6 Meal Plan

The next step I took was the 12-6 meal plan in my third through fifth years. I was able to make some significant progress in my weight-management during this time, and I felt a lot more energetic. In this plan, you have the same structure of an 8-6 meal plan, but you add an extra 4 hours to your fasting. During my work week, I would do this fasting routine. Instead of eating breakfast, I would drink 2 cups of coffee to start the morning. With this plan, I would be eating between the hours of 12pm and 6pm, with a full 18 hours of fasting during a period of 24 hours.

Although I was skipping breakfast, I knew that I needed to still drink a ton of water. The first time I tried this method, I failed to give myself enough water or fluids, and I had a terrible cramp and headache during the fast. It was rough. I also had to take some herbal tea to make me feel even more hydrated during my day. Because I had increased my fasting period, I needed to add even more fats to my diet; therefore, because I had a burger during that 8-6 window, I was able to add even more energy to my plan. It was amazing. Besides, I also saw myself adding more fruits and snacks that were high in fat content to be consumed around 3pm. Around dinner time at 6pm, I kept on with the meal plan that I did before with the 8-6, but then I would fast for an even more extended period.

The 12-6 plan was going to help me achieve my weight loss goals. I gained a little bit of fat on my bones over the years and had some problem with my muscle mass but, once I started this plan, I noticed that I was able to burn more fat and then that flab that I had on my belly was disappearing, and I knew that it was doing me good.

3. The 2-day Plan

Then, around year 5, I wanted to change everything up and wanted to modify my fasting. I knew that I wanted to take a rest from all the fasting and eat just a little bit on certain days. I also had lost weight over time and needed to keep on some pounds, as I was trying to gain muscle mass. So, what I did was do a modified plan, where I would eat anything I wanted to on five days, and then, for two days, I would only eat about 500 calories for those days. On the days where I wasn't fasting, I had to make sure I was getting enough fats, protein, fruits, and vegetables, among other things, to get my daily intake of essential nutrients. On the fasting days, I chose to eat smaller meals or snacks throughout the day, and then I would eat only some meat and cheese without bread for those days. I used some health and wellness apps to make sure I didn't go over 500 with the caloric intake.

This plan made it a little tougher for me. I started to have cramps and would get headaches because I was eating so little on a few days of my week. Then, I would binge on calories, fat, and carbs on my non-fasting days. It ended up being a bit complicated, and I was not happy with the overall result. This plan was harder to get right, so I wouldn't recommend it, except for the more advanced person to do, because it is going to be quite difficult some days. You should also consult a doctor before trying this kind of plan because it can be hard on your system. If you are taking medication, then it could be dangerous to engage in this type of fasting; therefore, you should exercise caution when trying out this way of fasting.

4. The 5-2 Plan

In this plan, I decided that I would eat for five days and do no eating for two days that are not in a row. For example, I would fast on Monday and Wednesday, but eat as usual on the other days of the week. On the five days, I would eat the same kinds of foods as before, including high-fat content, protein from meats, and fruits and veggies. I tried out this routine when I was in about years 6 and 7, and it was effective, but I would get hungry a lot more easily, as I think my body was burning at a faster rate. Combine this with an intensive workout, and you get a result that is losing weight and muscle mass; therefore, I would only recommend this fasting to someone who is well into their fasting routine after a few years of having done it. The method of fasting is not for beginners and can cause health problems if you are not careful. Please exercise caution with this one, as well.

5. Every-other-day Plan

This method of fasting proved to be one that provided breakthroughs in my life. I only resorted to it after the first seven years of doing fasting. It allowed me to build muscle power and stamina. My workouts were much better. I got sore less throughout the week, and I was able to recover from my workouts, as well. It helped so much. I also saw that I was ready to go for more extended periods without eating. I don't recommend this type of plan for beginners. You're going to have to wait a long time before you have the stamina for this plan because you will have to go for days without food throughout the week. You alternate the days that you fast, but you should still fill your diet with good meat and protein sources, good fats, fruits, and veggies. On the fasting days, you should drink lots of water and herbal tea, as well as some coffee and black tea. I would say that this one helped me a lot. If you're an experienced faster and you want to go the distance with your fasting, try this one out, but make sure you're getting the right foods into your system because you don't want to faint on the side of the street due to exhaustion. Proceed with caution.

The Warrior Diet

The final step in my journey to achieving the right balance with my dieting was the Warrior Diet. It is a type of intermittent fasting that includes a reduction of caloric intake for a period of time. It is based on the concept of warriors who ate very little during the day while they were on the hunt for food, and then they feasted for dinner. Ori Hofmekler founded it in 2001. In this plan, you fast for 20 hours a day and then eat as much food as you want at night; however, during the 20-hour window, you should consume a small amount of dairy, including eggs, fruits, and veggies, as well as plenty of fluids, including coffee, tea, and water. Following this period, you can eat as much food as you want from any type within 4 hours; however, you shouldn't eat too many processed foods during that time.

To get started with this plan, I followed a rigid three-week plan that allowed me to get to the point where I wanted to be. I will write later about that in this chapter. When I did this plan, I burned lots of fat, was able to concentrate on my work, and got spikes of energy that were just too good. It was terrific, and I felt a huge difference. It was like I was on top of the world.

Now, because this plan is so extreme, there was no way I could keep doing it for every day. I had to alternate it. Some days I would do it and other days I wouldn't. I had to make sure I was drinking enough fluids on the fasting days because that would make it or break it. This plan also comes with some risks that you need to be aware of. One example is that it can lead to disordered eating, including binging, which is not good for anyone. It can cause a lot of health complications. Additionally, it can cause you to have fatigue, lightheadedness, constipation, and imbalances, making it very difficult for some people to deal with; therefore, you should do this type of fasting rarely, or only on special occasions.

Let me show you how I did a rigid three-week plan to get this thing started:

Week 1: "The Detox"

During this period, I drank vegetable juices, dairy products such as milk, cheese, and yogurt, and hard-boiled eggs for 20 hours per day. Once I got to the 4-hour eating period, I ate a large salad with a raspberry vinaigrette and lots of pinto beans, whole grain bread, plus some cheese and stir-fried vegetables. This created a balanced diet that did not involve binging or any other type of thing. There is a reason that this stage is called the "detoxing period," and it is a stage in which you don't want to do too much in the way of modifying your diet.

Week 2: Add Fat

During the second week, I would eat some apples and bananas, dairy products, hard-boiled eggs, and tomato juice for the first 20 hours. During the 4 hours, I would consume a massive salad with a balsamic vinaigrette and chicken breast, as well as stir-fried zucchini squash, plus some pinto beans. However, during this phase, I did not consume a lot of carbohydrates from whole grains or starches.

Week 3: Lose Fat

This third week was a time in which I loaded up on the carbs. On the first two days, I would eat foods high in carbs, then on days 3-4, I would eat foods that were high in protein, but low in carbs. Then, on days 5-6, I would eat foods that were high in carbs. Finally, on the last day or two, I would eat foods that would be high in protein, but low in carbs.

On the high-carb days, I would eat the same thing as before with 20 hours of eating vegetable juice, dairy products, hard-boiled eggs, and apples and bananas. During the 4 hour window, I would eat a large tuna salad with a vinaigrette and stir-fried vegetables, as well as one carb such as pasta, rice, or corn. On the low-carb days, I would eat the same thing as before with 20 hours of eating vegetable juice, dairy products, hard-boiled eggs, and dried fruits. During the 4 hour window, I would eat a salad with lots of raw veggies, plus a grilled chicken breast and some stir-fried zucchini. Finally, for dessert, I would have a mango smoothie.

My experience with this one was kind of hard. I tried it but, in the beginning, I would feel sluggish, and my energy level would be difficult to manage. I wanted to nap as soon as the day started and, also, working out was a nightmare the first week or so that I tried doing this. The first time I tried the warrior method, I was working out intensely, but my energy level was tanking as soon as I got back. Also, I was so freaking hungry that I wanted to gorge myself right after I hit the gym. I ended up drinking lots of coffee to fill up my energy reserves again. It was super difficult, and I started to lose motivation to work out anymore. As I went through it (it felt like hell for a few weeks), I was able to overcome the difficulty and gorge myself less. As soon as the 4 hour window started, I would stuff myself with steaks and pasta. Basically, I would eat the most unhealthy way possible. I would also eat a huge piece of cheesecake for dessert, and get a ton of fat into my system.

After a few weeks, I wanted to quit, and I got down on myself. I struggled with self-concept and wanted to give up, but then my trainer helped me to get my ass up and do some more lifting. I then managed and decided to do the Warrior Diet only every other week. It helped, and I saw some good positive results with my appetite and gained some muscle mass.

This type of workout is for the experts who have done the intermittent fasting routine for a while. I would not recommend it to beginners or intermediate-level fasters, because it requires discipline and withholding from going crazy during the overeating period of 4 hours. You may be tempted to eat whatever the heck you feel like during that time, and you might gorge yourself with fatty and high cholesterol foods. I don't think that gorging yourself is going to help out with weight loss or with adding muscle power to your routine.

It's hard to recommend this workout for people that want to have a healthy balance because it feels like you're doing a Thanksgiving-type feast every night, and I am sure that is not good. You might also not want to try eating a 3,000 calorie meal. That could be overkill. Be careful with this meal option and don't try it if you're just starting out. You should wait for a long time before you try it as an option because so many people do it the wrong way and they end up having a ton of problems. I don't want you to make costly mistakes that will destroy your motivation to continue. It is best to heed this caution. I'm warning you; this method is dangerous and to be used with the utmost care and discipline. I have tried to give you an example of how to responsibly handle those 4 hours for fasting. Follow the model with that type of food, and you will be in for a successful time.

Conclusion

To conclude this section, as you can see, there is a diet and meal plan for every stage of your journey with intermittent fasting. You can choose which plan to take, but I would urge you to begin with an 8-6 plan first, and then increase to a 16-8 plan because these plans can be easily built into your schedule and they don't cause too much disturbance in your daily living. While you may encounter some problems with them, you may be able to get used to it; however, it will take weeks, if not months or years to reap the benefits fully. Long-term weight loss will not happen unless you stick to it, so I would, therefore, advise you to stick to the plan religiously to get the best results. At the same time, you don't want to harm yourself in the process. If at any point you feel pain, you should stop fasting and eat something. Don't gorge yourself; give yourself a banana or a glass of warm milk.

Through each step of the process, you will notice how much easier it gets to do your fast. Your stomach will get used to it and allow you to feed on the right nutrients. Your body will store healthy fat in its system, to promote a good energy level to sustain you throughout your day. Also, be sure that you are staying hydrated all day long because there is nothing worse than going through a fast without drinking enough fluids - that means water, tea, coffee, Powerade/Gatorade, and fruit drinks.

Finally, I urge you to take action today. Your diet is going to be an essential part of helping you manage your weight, whether or not you choose to do intermittent fasting. You will need to make healthy decisions about what you will eat so that you don't overcompensate on the wrong things. I want you to be successful in this process. Take control of your diet and then choose a plan that will be best for you in the intermittent fasting process.

CHAPTER 8

(YEARS 5-6)

WORKOUT AND INTERMITTNET FASTING

In this chapter, I will show you how to develop a great body by forming a workout routine that will make you look like a hot dude or girl. This period was when I started integrating an organized workout routine into my plan, which was years 5-6. I will explain my story and then tell you how you can also accomplish this goal of having the body of your dreams.

As a young lad, I was really slim and skinny. You wouldn't believe how I looked before. I had a little bit of fat in my stomach from where I would not work out anything in my body. Honestly, I hated going to the gym. I didn't like other people watching me and looking at my body as I was running and struggling to work out on the treadmill or lift at the bench press. I was ashamed of my body and thought I would never measure up to other guys or their ability to lift over 200 pounds. As I went along with intermittent fasting in my fourth year, I realized that if I wanted to get healthier, I needed to buff up. So, in my fifth year, I hired a personal trainer who would help me to reach my goals of getting fitter. His name was Jamie, and he taught me a lot of things about how I could get better at my fitness.

Together, Jamie and I came up with a plan to increase my muscle mass. It was not easy at first because I had to focus on my diet and I had to add more protein and carbs to my diet to increase my weight. I had to add about 1,500 calories to my diet to do this, and it was not easy because I had to start eating once every 2 hours. Basically, I was scarfing down egg salad sandwiches and other things all day. I had to eat as much as possible to make sure that I wouldn't lose any weight.

The ways that we were going to increase my weight included going to the gym three times a week for weight training, and twice a week for endurance training. Three days a week - Monday, Wednesday, and Friday - I would go to the gym to do strength training to focus on building my biceps, triceps, and other muscles. In between those days, I would rest, and then I would do no work on the weekends. The key was to do short intensive strength training exercises. In between, I would relax my muscles and eat a lot. The key would become how I would eat and rest because those are the times that are the most extended. You have to take advantage of all that time that you're not working out and do your best to maintain that.

Exercising While Fasting

Exercising when fasting is an integral part of your wellness routine, but you have to watch out because it can come with risks. Some research has shown that exercising when you fast can cause insulin sensitivity and the control of blood sugar levels. This is important to keep in mind if you have diabetes, which I have. When you exercise while fasting, you will likely burn more fat that will make your workout harder, but you may also lose muscle mass while using up a lot of protein. That could deplete your system, and you will have less energy, so you have to be very careful.

When you're fasting, you will burn more fat, which will enable you to lose weight while burning more fat. You may also lose a lot of energy by working this way, and you might not perform at your best. Also, you might lose muscle mass in the process, which will hinder your ability to build the muscle that you want.

The Solution to Dealing with the Challenges

When you're planning to work out while fasting, there are some considerations you should make. First, you should think about exactly when you will do the workout. One popular method is to use the 16-8 window, wherein you will do all your eating within 8 hours and fast for 16 hours. For better performance, it is best to plan your workouts within this 8 hour window, because then you will have the fuel that will keep you going for a length of time.

Secondly, you should choose a suitable type of workout based on the timing of your meals. You want to have a higher carb diet on days that you do your strength training, but you could do an endurance training day on days with low carbs.

Thirdly, if you work out, you need to plan on replenishing your body with energy and protein immediately upon completing your workout.

The main things to keep in mind is that you need to eat close to the time when you are doing your high-intensity workouts, and you need to drink lots of water and energy drinks to keep your body going through all aspects of the training. You should drink Gatorade or Powerade to have a higher electrolytes level. Also, with the intensity of the workout, you should keep it short and simple to avoid strain or injury that could come from working out too hard.

Finally, you need to listen to your body. If you feel hungry, eat. Don't allow your body to go for too long without food. When you exercise while fasting, undoubtedly, you will become hungrier with each passing minute. It is crucial that you get all the intake of calories and carbs in as soon as this happens because you will need to replenish the protein that is lost during intensive workouts. Also, make sure to include periods of rest in your routine that will enable you to do recover from intense workout cycles that can cause trauma to your system.

My Example

As I began my workout, I decided that I wanted to gain muscle mass. I was unsure how to go about it because I hadn't worked on it before. My personal trainer put me on a workout plan, and he worked with me on how to gain muscle mass, and we co-ordinated my meals around my workout times. I would work out in the afternoon just right before dinner so that I would be able to eat a high carb and protein meal with over 2,000 calories right away. That would immediately replenish all the protein I had lost during the workout, and then, I would eat less the next day in between workouts. I would always eat, work out, replenish and do this continuously to get the results that I desired. It worked for me.

Within a few months, I was able to build muscle mass. I gained 10lbs and could see the results in my biceps as I could see that there was some definition that was developing there. I was satisfied and thanked my personal trainer for helping me.

How It Can Help You Lose Weight

Because you may be eating during the cycles that you work out, you will lose some weight in the process while burning fat. It may be hard to do at first, but you have to time it just right. If your goal is to lose fat, then a good way is to time your workouts around the time of your fast but, then again, you might lose muscle mass, so be careful. Likewise, it is a good idea to do your workout during your time of eating, because your metabolism will get a boost of energy and you will see that you want more food; therefore, you will burn more calories and get a good result.

Conclusion

To sum up, working out while fasting is a great idea and can come with many benefits, but you also have to watch out and make sure you're not overdoing it. Also, you have to time your workouts at the right time and to replenish the energy that you will lose while working out. You don't want to get light-headed, dizzy, or have a headache from overdoing working out on an empty stomach. It is never a good idea. Be sure to take good care of yourself at all times so that you don't cause this problem. It is never a good idea to overdo the workout just so that you can lose a couple of pounds. You will develop a lot more risks and, potentially experience hazards that could be very dangerous for your health.

Once you decide on a good workout plan with a personal trainer or a trusted friend, you will be able to develop a useful framework for working out safely and effectively. Develop a game plan and stick to it, along with a diet that will work wonders for your overall health. Finally, have confidence that you are meant to achieve your dreams and goals in your health. All things are possible when you can carefully plan your future with achievable goals, so believe that it is possible. I know you can do it.

CHAPTER 9

(YEARS 7-10)

BENEFITS I AM SEEING IN MY BODY

In this chapter, I am going to highlight to you how I saw benefits in my body, work, relationships, and family. Intermittent fasting made a massive difference in my life, and I want to share with you how it all came about.

Before I started on this journey, I suffered from acid reflux, which also caused me to have "freaking heartburn." It happened after eating spicy food, but it also happened when I ate anything with fat or protein. My esophagus would burn like Hades, and I would have to go to the bathroom many times a day. It was so miserable. I went to the doctor and had to take heartburn pills for my acid reflux. One time I even had to go to the emergency room for having heart palpitations after eating a spicy Korean kimchi soup. It was horrible. I got out soon after that, but it was also at that point that I realized that I needed to take control of my health and what I ate. I would sometimes feel a terrible aching stomach pain that wouldn't go away unless I took medication for the condition. Day in, day out, I was going to the doctor for heartburn pain and feeling freaking miserable all the time. It was so hard, and I knew that I needed to get some help for it. The bloating and gas problem was a continual problem that I struggled with before doing intermittent fasting, as well.

After I decided to undertake the intermittent fasting in my third year, I started to notice the difference with my body. It took a while to get to this point, but I no longer felt like I had a bloating sensation. I no longer had a heaviness in my stomach every time I would eat something spicy. I was able to enjoy all the Korean and Indian food that my heart desired because I was able to take care of myself. I didn't have as much gas and the tendency to let it out at times, which was good, because my farts stank so much afterwards. It had to do with what I was eating, but also was due to the heartburn problem. I felt and looked better. No more of that sour feeling in my esophagus as soon as I downed a spicy chilly pepper from the Mexican restaurant. I felt loads better in what I could eat. I also was able to go to the bathroom easier. It made a big difference.

With my body, I could see and feel a tangible difference. I looked and felt great. I had a lot more energy from intermittent fasting and workouts. I was able to get the rest that I needed every night, and slept better as a result. Consequently, I got up every morning with a new sense of energy and determination to "seize the day." I was so excited to go to work and complete the projects that I had. Into my fifth year in the program, I enrolled in a financial advisor course at the local university. Within six months, I got my financial advisor license. I started working at an office in the downtown area and was making more money. I started making 50K per year and gradually increased my salary above that. I eventually was able to move out of my parents' house and rent my own place in the center of downtown LA. I bought a Ferrari and was able to score the job of my dreams. After I turned 34, I was really living it up and feeling prosperous as a young, single male. I enjoyed my singleness as a great time in my life.

I credit all this goal achievement to my discipline in doing this fasting routine. It made a huge difference. I knew that I needed to do all these things because I believed in myself. I also wanted to set high goals and objectives for myself because I knew I could accomplish more. My self-esteem increased over time, and then I knew that I could do all the things that I set my mind to because I had the discipline and willpower to get it done.

Additionally, my relationship with my parents improved. I enjoyed going home and talking to my mom and dad. I had a more positive attitude while talking to them and enjoyed helping them around the house. They were also more accommodating and welcoming to my new intermittent and workout schedule. Mom, especially, was happy to see that I had a healthy appetite. When I was younger, I used to be a very picky eater. I didn't enjoy eating fruit and vegetables, and my parents are vegan, so it helped that we were able to tackle this problem through the intermittent fasting. My parents saw me eating more healthily, and they wanted to help me with buying my food. They even got some fresh ingredients for me to cook at home. Mom let me help her with the gardening, and we grew some fresh tomatoes.

When I turned 35, I finally decided that I wanted to start dating. I was a shy guy and didn't want to be in a relationship. I was too self-conscious of my lean body and didn't want to have a girlfriend. As soon as I started working out and building muscle mass, I noticed that my testosterone level started going up and I became more interested in women, and then I realized that I wanted to date a woman. I started picking up women and dated several girls. It was hard at first, and I got my heart broken a couple of times but, when I reached age 36, I found the girl of my dreams. Her name was Rachel, and she was terrific. We immediately understood each other. She was attracted to me because I was a goal-oriented and hardworking man. We went out for a few months and, in the summer of that year, I got engaged to her. It was awesome.

As you can see, this intermittent fasting routine helped me so much, and I got to meet different people and finally met my wife-to-be. After doing the method for a while, I got out of my singleness and aspired for more. I wanted to become a husband. It changed my life priorities, and I realized that I had to aspire to be great and to achieve what had been seemingly impossible before.

What All This Means for You

If you're reading this, then you know that you have to take action. You can't just sit on your ass and do nothing about it. You have to get out there and do it. You've got to get out there and do your thing, and that means that you can also get the body that you desire with the muscle mass that you want. You are going to have to set goals for yourself and schedule the time to do all the things you need to do. Schedule your fast, watch your diet and you will be able to accomplish your goal. You should also put that picture of yourself, that you want to be, on your mirror. Maybe that's a Hugh Jackman or Tom Cruise picture. Imagine yourself with that six pack and huge biceps, and then, get 'er done. Go to the gym. Go swimming. Lift weights. Do all that is necessary to build up your physique. Eat like crazy for 8 hours during your day - once every hour or two. Snacking also helps you. Engage in your physical exercise.

If you follow through with all the things above, then you can start building muscle mass, and then fast and rest. Enjoy the time when you're not eating or doing activities. Rest is so crucial to your wellbeing. Believe that you can do it. It won't be easy. You might be tired and frustrated a lot of the time. I know I felt like shit sometimes and wanted to quit. I got so tired of not eating and was so tempted to break the fast and eat a bag of Cheetos while watching Grey's Anatomy re-runs. Believe me, I've been there. It felt like rock bottom and was freaking depressing. What I am saying is that it is worth all of it, because you can go for that goal with all your might and achieve the body of your dreams, because you have envisioned it in your heart.

Conclusion

To conclude, I think that it is essential to keep in mind continually your goal and the body you want to get. Having a mental picture of the man that you want to be is important because you have to strive and do your best to achieve it. Don't think for a second that it won't involve you stretching yourself, because if you think it's a smooth ride and you can sit on your ass and vedge on Netflix every day, then you're in for a hard time. I'm not going to lie to you. It's going to suck sometimes. You're going to want to cry and sulk when you can't reach for that gallon of ice cream after 6pm and eat your feelings. You're going to ache and groan from the pain of not taking in any calories. You might have a headache. Heck, you might fall flat on your face because you haven't eaten in 15 hours. I've been there. I know the pain. It sucks but, once you've reached your breaking point, you will realize how strong of a man you are. You know that you have overcome so much in your life. This was one small inkling of a time when you had to endure and, no matter how painful as shit this time is, you know that you will be able to achieve your dream and that makes you want to celebrate your achievement. Do it because you care about yourself. Do it because you want to be a better man. Do it so that you can get the ladies to come and go out with you.

I was successful with it, and I know that you can be, too. Hang in there friend, I know you can do it. It's going to be hard, but once you've accomplished it, there will be a wave of euphoria that will change your life. This is going to be a long road to the finish line. It took me ten years to get where I am, but every step of the way made a difference and I am a better man as a result. I believe you can do it too, so let's do this thing!

CHAPTER 10

THE MAN I AM TODAY (10 YEARS LATER)

Here I am. It is my 38th birthday, and I am 10 years into this intermittent fasting journey. There's been a lot of heartache through these years. I now want to tell you where I am at after these ten years and what my dreams and hopes are for the future, as well as pointers for you to have.

I've already told you about how I started this journey with no ambition and only wanted to get by and pay my bills and live in my parents' basement. Since starting the journey, I moved out of my parents' house, got my own place and lived alone for a while, got an fantastic job and a great car and house, and then got married. All these things happened over time as I wanted to achieve each milestone. Not bad for a man who had no ambition, right?

The point I have wanted to get across to you in this book is that you have to have some ambition to get where you want to be. You must set a target and goal for yourself. I was able to do that every step of the way while approaching each part of the journey with care and dedication. It was a lot of hard work and blood, sweat, and tears. There were moments where I sat on the toilet and was crapping a boatload because I had an upset stomach from working out too much and not eating enough. Those headaches would hurt like shit, and I found myself dazed and confused at times. Sometimes, I struggled with insomnia because of hunger pains. As we saw before, I had a series of struggles and mistakes that I made that were difficult for me. At the end of the ten years, I made it through. I went through all the meal plans that I have described in detail. I did the 8-6, 16-8, the 5-2, and the warrior plan for several years, alternating between plans each month and year.

I will be honest with you. I struggled a lot with motivation on my own. I needed accountability. That's why I talked to my trusted friend and trainer Jamie. We worked together throughout those years, and Jamie became like a best friend to me. We enjoyed hanging out together frequently, and we eventually got to go traveling together to Europe and Asia. I opened up to Jamie about my struggles. I would highly recommend that you also find a trusted friend to reach out to in this process. There's no way to go on this journey alone; you need to have accountability. Trust me on this point.

In all my time, I have needed not only the support of my trusted friend and trainer, but also my friends and family. Over time, people became kinder and supportive of the kind of efforts I was making. People no longer made fun of me. They saw the difference to my body that this fasting was making. They saw the six-pack and muscle definition that I was getting over time. Men and women were admiring my body, and I knew that it was making a difference. People became attracted to me and my positivity. I was glowing with pride every time I'd talk about intermittent fasting and how it had changed my life. They also felt like they could relate to my story because it is relevant and makes people think about their own lives. I knew that this journey had started and ended with some good fodder to help others get started with their journey.

So, I have to ask you, are you ready to begin? I want you to be prepared for a transformation, and I want to give you all the tools and tips that will help you successfully launch your intermittent fasting training plan. You've seen what a difference it has made in my life. I believe it can also happen in your life. I am excited to share some of the powerful tips that you can use to begin the adventure of your life. It's not only going to be for a year or two; it's going to be the adventure of a lifetime. You will make decisions and cultivate habits that will follow you for the rest of your life. I know, because I am going to use the habits I have formed through this process for a very long time. It's ingrained into who I am.

Let's do this thing. Read on to find out about the tips that will help you to get started in the next and final chapter of the book.

CHAPTER 11

POWERFUL TIPS TO MAKE YOU START NOW

As you have seen so far in this book, intermittent fasting changed my life. It has a host of benefits that have made me more confident in myself and have led me to pursue a life of greatness, which is following my heart's desire to get lean and fit. Over the past ten years, many people have wanted to know more about intermittent fasting and its popularity. Intermittent fasting has many benefits that include weight loss, reversing type 2 diabetes, savings in time and money, among others.

In this chapter, we are going to show you how you can get the most out of your fasting routine. Let's begin with the basics:

How Long Do You Want to Fast?

24-hour Fasts

This is a way of fasting from dinner to dinner (or lunch to lunch). For example, if you eat dinner on the first day, you would not eat breakfast the next day or lunch and then eat dinner again the following day. In this case, you would be eating once daily. It would be recommended that you do this type of fast only two to three times per week. You can get the most benefits by doing this because you can replenish your energy one time per day and then fast for 24 hours. This is an effective means to do it.

My Example

I usually do this type of fasting once or twice a week. It has helped me to maintain my metabolism and restores my system after eating many heavy meals. It has helped me to keep a healthy weight and has given me some flexibility in varying my time spent in fasting.

5:2 Fast

This fast is done when you have five days where you eat regularly and two fasting days; however, on the fast days, you take in only 500 calories each day. You can consume these calories either all at once or spread out throughout the day.

My Example

Every two weeks, I do this type of fasting, and it helps me when I feel weak and need time to recharge my system. I have found that if I can take it easy on the fasting for a few days in a month, it helps me to do better, and I also don't have as many hunger pains in my system and a stomach ache that hurts terribly.

36-hour Fasts

During this fast, you would fast for the entire day. You would eat dinner on the first day, and then fast for the whole day of the second day, and then not eat again until day three at breakfast time. This type of fasting is used to promote weight loss. Also, it allows you not to be tempted to overeat on the second day.

My Example

I do this fast once a month, like when I want to do a spiritual retreat and meditate. I go up to a mountain and don't eat and spend some time reflecting and meditating. It is excellent, and I can truly connect with my feelings and emotions.

Shorter Fasts

Many people will do a 16-8 fast. In this fast, you do it for 16 hours, and then you eat within a window of 8 hours. During the eight hours, you consume all the nutrients in your system. To be honest, this is the fast that I do most of the time. It is something that Hugh Jackman once recommended, and I want to recommend it to you. For most people, this type of fast is totally possible and doesn't require much thought or effort on the part of the person fasting.

Within the eight hours, a person does not eat anything, and then a person will eat all his or her meals between 11:00 am and 7:00 pm. Many people choose to skip breakfast during this time, but others skip dinner and only eat breakfast and lunch.

In my case, I decided I wanted to do intermittent fasting by skipping breakfast. Instead of eating anything for breakfast, I decided to opt for something that many people in America want - coffee. It gets me through the day and allows me to wake up without having to overeat in the morning. And then I eat lunch and dinner. It saves me a heck of a lot of money, time, and energy to prepare breakfast, and I'd recommend that you try it as well.

There is also the 20-4 fast. During this time, you eat during a 4-hour eating window and then fast for 20 hours. I found that this method was not as effective, and I would often have a terrible headache by fasting for about twenty hours. I wouldn't recommend this one, as it did cause me a lot of problems.

What are Some of the Side Effects that I Might Encounter?

As with any diet plan, there are risks to consider, and you should consult a doctor or a trusted person who can guide you through this process. I am no doctor, so don't quote me on this information, but I think that it is crucial that you find a way of working with a professional, who can aid in different dietary and medical needs that you may have. If you are taking medication, I would strongly advise consulting a doctor, because who knows what might happen if you start fasting and then you have high blood pressure or some other result. You want to be careful.

Hunger: You will likely experience severe pain whenever you fast, and you might get a rumbling of your stomach during lunch, which may continue for a long time. Those hunger groans may happen for a while, so you have to be careful. You may also have a stomach ache after not eating for a while.

Headaches: You may experience migraines or other problems that can be painful to endure. It will be hard on your system, and you might seriously want to quit the program at this point, but I would advise you to stick through it.

Constipation: Because you're not eating as much, you won't have to go to the bathroom as much, and it may make you less regular to go to the toilet. Try a laxative if you cannot go to the bathroom for an extended period.

Hazy feeling and lightheadedness: Whenever you do your intermittent fasting plus exercise, you will feel a bit light-headed so prepare for this, especially in the beginning. You're going to struggle with doing your day-to-day activities because it is brand new to you.

Low energy, especially in the beginning: When you start exercising and fasting, you will lose a lot of energy first, because your body is getting used to fasting and exercising. Be ready to handle this aspect.

Lack of motivation and a desire to quit: This is the one that we all will encounter at some point in our lives. There is a genuine desire to quit that you may experience when you're on this journey that you're going to have to be ready for. It will hit you like a red brick sometimes, so you're going to have to brace yourself for it before it affects you. While it is challenging at the start, it will get better with time.

Desire to binge when eating and do unhealthy things: One last point is that you want to avoid binging on foods, but it will be a temptation that you will inevitably have. When a person is hungry, he will want to vedge out, so you will have to learn how to deal with this side effect.

What Are Some of the Things to Keep in Mind During a Fast?

Stay hydrated. Drink lots of water during your intermittent fasting. I cannot stress this point enough. You have to drink as much water as possible because you have to take care of yourself. Your body is made up of mostly water, so you have to make sure you're getting enough water in your system daily. Don't ever skimp on this point. You can also be hydrated by ways other than just water;

for example, you could drink energy drinks or other things like that. The important thing is not to do too much activity without water or other beverages. This is especially the case if you are exercising or working out a lot.

Keep a busy schedule. Another thing you have to do is stay busy because this will make a difference in how you can live a good life. There is an old saying that says "Idleness is a devil's tool." I think that is true. You have to stay busy to get ahead in life. You cannot just sit on your ass all day, watch TV re-runs, and do other things. You have to do a lot of things in your life. Enjoy socializing with others. Have a life. Get ahead in your career. There are a lot of things that I would recommend you to do. You have to make the most of every moment, because the thing is, this life is short. You've got to get a lot out of it and make a meaningful life, and that does not mean sitting around and doing nothing and waiting for someone to tell you what to do. It means having a game plan and sticking to it. This will help you to enjoy your fasting more. You will not even notice that you took the time out of your schedule to fast because you will be so busy doing all the things that make a difference in the world.

Have a cup of coffee or tea. This point is so important. Tea and coffee are filled with antioxidants and are useful to help you have more energy, and we know that caffeine is what keeps most of the world going. Coffee also has a natural appetite suppressant that enables you to go for longer without eating anything.

Keep trying, don't give up. I would also recommend that you keep trying and do not give up because the plan should be in place, such that you will achieve your goal, whether that is weight loss or some other plan, so keep doing it. You can do it! I believe you can. Trust me. It's hard, and it will take some hard work, but it is worth everything for you to achieve that body that you deserve to have.

Don't eat too much after fasting. One thing that you definitely should avoid is binging after you fast. If you do a fast, you should avoid having a feast the day you stop. Not a good idea, believe me, been there, done that. I vomited up a storm after it. Horrible. Never again. I would highly recommend that you do not overeat. Don't go out to Cracker Barrel or the Golden Corral following an extended period of fasting.

Break the fast gradually. This point goes with #5. You have to be gradual with resuming your regular dieting. It is crucial that you return with a little bit at a time, rather than overloading your system, which can lead to complications and difficulties. You don't want to shock your system with food and cause stomach pain or other abdominal conditions.

Who Shouldn't Fast?

Another point we need to go over is who are the people who shouldn't fast. First, if you are underweight and have a low BMI, it is highly recommended that you don't fast. Also, pregnant women should not try intermittent fasting. Finally, people that are involved in intensely athletic activities, such as team sports, should take care not to fast because of the high energy that is exerted within those activities.

How to Begin Now

Ok, so now you have decided to do intermittent fasting. Congratulations! You're ready to embark on this fantastic adventure that you will not regret that you did. I know that you have looked at many case studies in this book of how I was able to use intermittent fasting and it changed my life. I am no longer the same man. I think that you can also do the same thing. So, if you're committed to seeing your life change, let's begin now. Here are the action steps that I would recommend you take in the coming days:

Decide on what type of fast you want to do. Is the 16-8 fast ideal for your schedule? What about the 5-2 fast? The 24-hour fast? Think about which option you want to do. You should carefully consider which one fits your needs, body type, and goal, etc.

Decide how long it will be for. Will this fast be for one week, two weeks, or longer? Choose a duration for your program, and how long you will do it. Often, our bodies are created to do some activity for a period of time, but in brief spurts. Think of when you were studying 8 hours a day for final exams when you were in college. The same principle applies here, so choose a duration that is appropriate for your project.

Start fasting! Now that you have planned your fast, do it! You can do it! It will be amazing. It will be tough, and you may want to quit, but you have to carry out your project and do it with passion.

Continue doing your everyday activities as usual. Even when you're fasting, you can continue doing your day-to-day activities as you did before. It will take time to get used to it; however, you will need to make your system adjust.

Break the fast at an appropriate time. After this, you should break your fast gradually, and without binging or having a feast so that you won't get sick.

Repeat your fast within a designated period.

Conclusion

Now that you have an excellent resource from my experience and knowledge, you can use it to start your own intermittent fasting plan. Follow the steps and method that I have outlined for you with the tips, and you will be able to see the results you want to see. The main thing you need to do is have a game plan that you can stick to. It needs to have a clear and achievable goal that you can use. Choose your fast, the duration, and how you will do it. Schedule your meals. Keep in mind the precautions and warnings that we have highlighted here. Be careful and take the right measures to protect your health. If you feel unbearable pain, you should stop fasting and eat something right away. We don't want you to do something dangerous to your health. Take good care of yourself. You can and will succeed if you follow our detailed instructions, and I am a living testimonial to how it has worked for me.

CONCLUSION OF CHAPTERS

To wrap up what we have talked about, I want to inspire you to think big about your life. We only live maybe 70 or 80 years at most on average, and we have to get the most out of our lives. I want you to live an amazing life that is filled with joy, peace, and prosperity. I don't want you to waste your time trying to figure out a strategy that may or may not work from a fancy expensive diet plan. What I have offered you is a simple solution that has positive and significant results with intermittent fasting.

I was a shy, lanky man before, who had no kind of physique before starting a diet and intermittent fasting plan. As I said in the introduction, I had no plan for my life, no way going forward because I was so focused on fleeting pleasures. I was going to lose out on so many things because I was not paying attention to my health. Learning about my diabetes diagnosis and my mom's death from cancer, I felt that I needed to take the necessary steps to protect my health, because, the truth is, it's a gift to have good health. No-one is entitled to it. If you're lucky enough to not get sick in a year, then you are living a good life.

Don't you want to live a life filled with good health? Don't you want to have a hot body that everyone wants? Do you want to have a girlfriend or boyfriend that you know you deserve? Look no further than intermittent fasting. It is a proven technique that works. Many celebrities, including Hugh Jackman, have endorsed it and use it regularly. If you can make intermittent fasting part of your diet routine, you may see some sustained and extensive results to your weight management plan, and you may be able to lose the weight that you have now.

Don't think for a moment that it is going to be easy. I have already enumerated the struggles, pain, and anxiety that I had to go through to get where I am now. It took a lot of difficulty and challenges to arrive at the point where I am today. I couldn't get through it without the support of my parents, friends, trainer, and my wife. All my loved ones eventually jumped on the bandwagon and supported me in all the efforts that I made. That has made the most significant difference in my life; therefore, I urge you to get the kind of support system that is going to allow you to achieve the results that you desire. It's going to be hard to do it on your own; I would say, impossible. No person can operate on their own. Everyone needs someone else to help them. We're meant to live our lives in community with one another. That means supporting the weaker person and encouraging them. You need someone to cheer you on the race to the finish line. Life is a marathon; you've got to pace yourself and have your cheerleaders to back you up when the going gets tough.

As you go through this journey, I recommend you look back at this small book of tips, experience, and ideas for inspiration. Remember the struggles that I have highlighted to you. Recall the adventure that it was for me. There were some fantastic victories that I experienced, and I was so glad to reach different milestones throughout my life. I believe that with patience, hard work, endurance, and perseverance, it is absolutely possible for you to achieve the milestones that you have set for yourself in your own life.

Here is my last call to action. Get out there. Do your thing. Start exercising. Go to the gym and get on an exercise plan. Run laps, swim in the pool, do whatever floats your boat and find some muscle exercises that will strengthen your core. Choose a workout plan and meal plan that will enable you to do the fasts that you want to do to get the results. Stick to your project like a religion. You have to be consistent if you're going to see the results that you want. Hang in there when the going gets tough; it won't always be easy. You may be excited at the beginning of the journey, but that excitement will wane over time. You still have to keep going. Keep your eye on the prize - whether that is to lose weight, gain muscle mass, or just live a healthy lifestyle.

VL DEALEXANDER

Intermittent Fasting for Weight Loss

Complete Guide to Transforming Your Body in 15 Days or Less Guaranteed!

<u>Meal Plan Included</u>

VL DeAlexander

CONTENTS

1   Introduction   1

2   Understanding Intermittent Fasting   4

    Why Do People Use Intermittent Fasting

    The Science Behind Intermittent Fasting

    How You Can Use Intermittent Fasting to Lose Weight

    Other Possible Benefits of Intermittent Fasting

    Common Myths and Issues with Intermittent Fasting

3   Types of Intermittent Fasting   24

    The Daily Method, Also Known as Leangains

    The Warrior Method

    Alternately Eating: Eat Stop Eat

    Fat Loss Forever Method

    Alternate Day Fasting

4   Losing Weight with Intermittent Fasting   31

    Example Meal Plan for Weight Loss with Intermittent Fasting

Exercising with Intermittent Fasting

5   Can You Build Lean Muscle with Intermittent   41
    Fasting?

6   Developing an Intermittent Fasting Meal Plan   47

    Examples of Meal Plans for 16/8 Intermittent
    Fasting Option

    Planning Your Meals for Specific Goals

    Calculating Your Daily Macro Requirements

7   Tips for Getting Started with Intermittent Fasting   59

    Here Is a Step-By-Step Guide to Help You Out

    Apps and Tools That Will Make Your Journey
    Easier

8   Who Should Avoid Intermittent Fasting?   63

9   The Scientific Evidence Behind Intermittent Fasting 66

10 Frequently Asked Questions About Intermittent   76
    Fasting

11 Conclusion   84

    References   87

CHAPTER 1

INTRODUCTION

Obesity has become a serious problem all over the world. The World Health Organization has recently announced that since the year 1975, the prevalence of obesity has increased by 300%. Over 650 million people are estimated to be obese throughout the world – and up to 1.9 billion people are also estimated to be overweight.

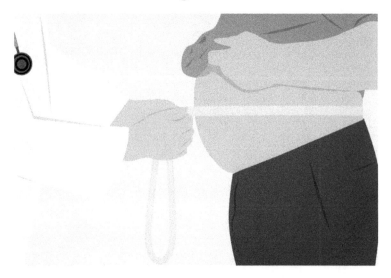

The health risks that obesity carries are serious issues. A number of diseases such as type 2 diabetes, hyperlipidemia, metabolic syndrome, cancer and coronary heart disease, high blood pressure, which can lead to stroke, originate from carrying an excessive amount of body fat. Let's take a look at how obesity has led to some of the diseases mentioned above.

- **Coronary heart disease** - being overweight means that the body mass index (BMI) rises. With obesity, the arteries that supply blood to the heart thicken due to the build-up of a sticky substance called plaque which can hinder blood flow and cause a heart attack.
- **High blood pressure** - the power by which the heart pumps blood through the veins and arteries is known as blood pressure. Obesity causes an increase in this pressure, which leads to many problems in the body over time.
- **Stroke** – obesity, as previously mentioned, causes the formation of plaque. Over time this plaque can cause the formation of blood clots called thrombus. A detached clot causes many serious problems throughout the body: myocardial infarction or heart attack if it lodges in the heart, pulmonary embolism if it travels to the lungs, and stroke if the clot lodges in the brain. Each one is a medical emergency that can be fatal.
- **Abnormal blood fats** – being overweight usually causes an in-crease in bad cholesterol in the body, causing a decrease in good cholesterol.

High cholesterol is bad for health and is a risk factor for illness caused by coronary heart disease

Women who are pregnant may also experience problems with their pregnancy due to the complications that obesity causes them to experience.

To address the worldwide prevalence of obesity, a significant number of diets, supplements, and programs have been released. These programs aim to help obese individuals lose the excess weight they have gained, with the hopes of restoring their optimal health. While some of these diets have shown impressive results, even when studied in clinical trials, many do not work, cause people to gain more weight in the long run, and even lead to side-effects.

Intermittent fasting is a type of lifestyle change that many people have adopted recently. Many tend to confuse this "lifestyle option" with a diet – it is not exactly a diet that a person needs to follow, but rather a way of eating – scheduling of food consumption is the most important part of this lifestyle plan.

Here, we will introduce you to intermittent fasting. We'll consider what intermittent fasting really is, the different types of this "dietary" or "lifestyle" option that is available, how it works, and we will, of course, also consider the benefits and possible drawbacks that everyone should be aware of before setting out to implementing this "eating pattern" into their lives.

CHAPTER 2

UNDERSTANDING INTERMITTENT FASTING

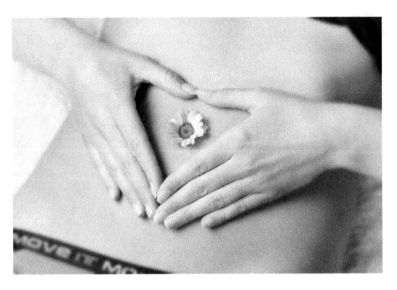

Let us start by taking a look at what intermittent fasting is. The term has become quite popular in recent years, but there is still a lot of confusion in regards to what this term really means and what it involves. Many people think that the term "intermittent fasting" refers to a diet, but this not actually a diet. Instead, it is rather an eating habit that people adopt that gives them guidance on when they should eat – this allows the digestive system to take a break from processing and digesting food continuously.

For many people, this type of dietary habit seems unhealthy. There is a lot of people who are scared of adopting this pattern of eating because they think that they would starve themselves. This, however, is a com-mon myth that has been told about intermittent fasting.

This particular dietary scheduling technique has been used since ancient times. Numerous scientific studies have been conducted to determine how the technique interacts with the human body, and several ad-vantages have already been noted.

An important fact that you should know when it comes to discussing this method of eating is that, since it is not classified as a diet, it will not decide the types of food that you will be eating. It is up to you to decide what you want to eat. A healthy, balanced diet that is filled with foods high in essential nutrients will, of course, result in more benefits as com-pared to stuffing yourself with hamburgers and pizza as soon as the clock strikes five, or whatever time it is your eating cycle starts. When opting for fast foods and other food options that are very high in carbohydrates, weight loss may not be a particular benefit that you experience when following this diet.

Why Do People Use Intermittent Fasting?

There are many different reasons why people use the intermittent fasting technique. These techniques date back to ancient times – they were used historically for a number of different purposes. For example, in older times, when a village would be limited to their food supply, people in the village would often implementing a type of fasting technique to help make the food last longer. Careful planning had to go into such a technique as the villagers had to eat enough food to support their bodily functions, at the right times, while still ensuring the inventory of available food could last until more food would become available.

Certain religions also have certain celebrations and festivals where people fast. Religions that incorporate fasting include Buddhism, Judaism, Islam, Hinduism, Bahai, Jainism, Raelism, and Sikhism. Certain types of Christian religions also use fasting for various purposes. This includes Catholicism, Orthodoxy, Mormonism, and Protestantism. These religions use fasting in different ways, and the technique serves a different purpose in each religion. Some religions also only utilize parts of these fasting techniques and will not completely eliminate all foods from a per-son's diet for a set period of time.

Many people also tend to go on a fast when they

feel sick, whether they have contracted the flu or another type of disease. This is because food does not work well with nausea and vomiting, nor with other types of gastrointestinal symptoms.

In modern times, however, more-and-more people are starting to adopt an intermittent fasting lifestyle – often not because they are sick or be-cause of religious requirements, but rather due to the health benefits that have been associated with this scheduled eating habit.

While weight loss is surely the most popular benefit that tends to be the reason why people usually opt for intermittent fasting, it is important to realize that there are more benefits that can be achieved as well. In particular, it has been found that this technique actually changes certain cells in the body. This, in turn, can cause changes in human growth hormone regulation, insulin regulation, and even improve the body's ability to re-pair cells.

Fasting has also been linked to reductions in low-grade chronic inflammation throughout the body, lower levels of oxidative stress in body tis-sues and cells, as well as potential improvements in a person's cardiovascular health. In turn, this combination of powerful benefits may lead to a longer lifespan – while this has not been proven yet, long-term studies are currently being conducted to see whether these benefits can, in fact, prolong a person's life.

The Science Behind Intermittent Fasting

Understanding how exactly intermittent fasting work is one of the essential elements that need to be covered before you dive into it and start adopting this method of eating in your own life. By learning more about how it works, you can get a better idea of whether or not this might be a good option for you – and if you would be able to benefit from it truly.

This eating habit basically involves cycles of eating and abstaining from food. There are different techniques and methods that have been introduced over the last few years, so not everyone will follow this lifestyle option in the same way as others. Generally, however, all options that are available involved periods of time where food is consumed, and then periods where the person would completely avoid eating any type of food.

When eating normally, with three meals a day and in-between snacks, the body uses energy from the recently consumed meal first, seeking out carbohydrates (CHO) and sugars, which it prefers to burn before anything else. Without intermittent fasting, normal persons (non-diabetics) insulin sensitivity will be at normal levels, and will detect stored glycogen at "full level." With sufficient blood glucose levels, excess energy will be stored as fat. If this happens on a regular basis, the determinants for the difference in body weight will lie in the level of activity and metabolic rate which slows down with age, resulting in weight gain.

When on intermittent fasting, the body behaves

differently when food is present (feasting) and during the period of abstinence (fasting), as compared to normal eating. The body produces insulin in response to the presence of food, enabling the body to get the most from them, maximizing nutrients for optimum results. Since eating is confined to a desired set window of 4, 6, or 8 hours, the body will not have a ready source of energy during the fasted state and will tend to extract energy from stored fat rather than from glucose traveling in the blood or glycogen stored in the liver or muscles.

Insulin sensitivity is increased after a fast. We can illustrate this insulin sensitivity by analyzing the cascade of events that take place when such a person eats something. As blood glucose rises, it activates a feedback mechanism which signals the pancreas to send insulin to the site where it is needed. An immediate response serves to lower the blood glucose and prevent its accumulation in the blood, or hyperglycemia. Here, insulin responds with a "now you see it, now you don't" type of mechanism: a sharp peak in response to the rising blood glucose, followed by an immediate decline. This is documented by lower readings of 2-hour postprandial blood glucose and insulin measurements.

Diabetics, on the other hand, suffer from insulin resistance, wherein the pancreas secretes only small bursts of insulin in response to glucose, followed by a slowed decline, resulting in higher 2-hour postprandial blood glucose and insulin measurements.

How You Can Use Intermittent Fasting to Lose Weight

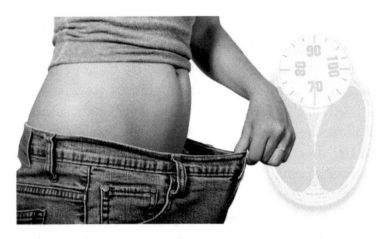

The majority of people who wishes to start implementing intermittent fasting into their lives want to do so due to the weight loss benefits that have been reported. It is well-known by now that this type of eating habit can help a person shed extra weight, primarily through the reduction of calories. Several scientific studies have also been conducted on this topic, and the results have been quite positive thus far. This is why we decided to look at the benefits that intermittent fasting may have for a person who is obese or overweight, and who is currently struggling to lose weight with conventional diets and other types of weight loss programs.

This eating pattern has two particular benefits that should be considered when it comes to losing weight. Firstly, it has been scientifically proven to help shed excess fat. This is a major advantage over traditional diets and dieting supplements – most programs, diets and even the pills that can be taken to initiate weight loss often tend to reduce weight through a reduction in "water weight." Rarely do they truly help a person lose actual fat? With intermittent fasting, however, science has proven that a person burns fat and their body fat percentage becomes reduced when they implement this technique into their lives and strictly stick to the particular routine they have decided on.

The other major benefit in regards to weight loss is that this scheduled eating plan has also been proven to preserve the lean muscle mass in a person's body while they lose weight. This is an important factor that needs to be taken into account. Lean muscle mass is important for several functions of the human body and also helps to make the movement more comfortable.

For example, lean muscle mass has been proven beneficial in the prevention of insulin resistance, as well as diabetes. A loss of lean muscle mass has also been associated with a higher incidence of illness. Cancer patients, for example, who loses muscle mass while undergoing treatment are less likely to survive and more likely to experience a recurrence of the disease should they survive, as compared to those who maintain healthier levels of muscle mass.

Furthermore, research has also been proven that lean muscle mass helps to maintain stronger bones.

When bones are kept in a healthy and strong state, then a person is less likely to experience problems such as fragile bones and problems maintaining their balance. The person will also be less likely to suffer an injury during physical activity. The risk of osteoarthritis and similar diseases are also lower among individuals with stronger bones and better levels of lean muscle mass.

Several suggestions have been made regarding the way that intermittent fasting would help a person lose excess fat, while also preserving their existing muscle mass. The effect that these scheduled eating habits have on the body's metabolism is thought to play a significant role here. For example, one review paper explains that the gut flora, often also called the microbiome, is affected by intermittent fasting. This, in turn, can help to improve metabolism and make the digestive system more efficient.

Another study explains that, even though it is widely recognized this that habit of eating based on specific cycles are beneficial for obese individuals, little data is available on how exactly this works on a biological or physiological level. The study found that fat reduction is possible primarily due to adipose thermogenesis that occurs due to the energy or caloric restriction imposes upon a person's body with this type of approach to eating.

Other Possible Benefits of Intermittent Fasting

Besides weight loss, intermittent fasting carries

with it many other health benefits, some of which are:

The practice of intermittent fasting is for every individual who is interested in the accrual of health benefits into his life. It is not designed merely for the obese or the out-of-shape clientele. Maintaining optimal health is both a privilege and responsibility of every human being created by God.

Intermittent fasting breeds longevity. Scientific studies have re-ported that this eating pattern results in positive outcomes in favor of improving quality of life. So it is not just staying alive per se, but being able to live and appreciate life fully. Imagine our body as a machine that undergoes wear and tears with the stress of eating, digestion, calorie utilization, delivery to the tissues and elimination of wastes. Intermittent fasting would cut that wear and tear right in the middle, because eating is confined within a personally chosen window, and the body is given a respite from the digestive processes during the fasting period.

Knowing that the human body is never idle, even during rest, and that there is always something going on inside, pathways are activated, signaling the body to quickly grab the opportunity to regenerate, repair and rejuvenate muscles, organs, and tissues, thereby delaying the aging process.

Intermittent fasting has the long-term effect of normalizing insulin sensitivity. This is beneficial because insulin resistance plays a crucial role in the etiology of chronic diseases such as Diabetes

Mellitus Type 2, Heart Disease and certain types of cancer.

Intermittent fasting curbs hunger by regulating the level of ghrelin, which is known as the "hunger hormone."

Intermittent fasting activates the Growth Hormone, which plays a pivotal role in overall health and muscle growing fitness.

Intermittent fasting reduces inflammatory conditions and promotes cellular resistance to free radical damage through the process of natural detoxification.

Intermittent fasting normalizes blood pressure and blood lipids.

Intermittent fasting simplifies the daily routine. Mothers no longer have to rush through the morning to prepare breakfast for the family, prepare and hustle the kids off to school, rush to the office if she is a working mom, and the list goes on. This is an interesting benefit that is attributed to intermittent fasting. We only have to plan for 1-2 meals a day depending on your chosen window, ideally composed of 30-35% high-quality chewable protein in the form of meat, 30-35% fat from non-animal sources, and 35-40% complex carbohydrates.

Intermittent fasting lowers the risk of cancer. The development of cancer on a cellular level is encouraged by the quality of food consumed, especially those high in sugars, saturated fat, seasonings, coloring, and preservatives, to name a few. Because intermittent fasting would require a dramatic change not only in the frequency of meals but also in the nutrient content, the body would be less subjected to assault from the toxins from highly processed food and empty calories. With restricted calories, our body has much more time to burn the food and optimize the use of nutrients, using up fat stores which are known to fuel breast and other reproductive organ cancers. Also, high fiber content would serve to mobilize and excrete any present undesirables out of the body. Another important caveat is, that cancer cells feed on sugars, while high fructose, an ingredient which is present in various forms, whether overt or covert, causes cancer cell division.

Intermittent fasting delays the aging process, especially if combined with some form of exercise. Stress resistance is enhanced, reducing oxidative damage up to the cellular level, acting as a deterrent to aging. Increased resistance against free radicals also discourages the development of inflammatory diseases and some forms of cancer. Also, studies have shown that fasting before chemotherapy increases the success rate of the treatment, as evidenced by the destruction of neuroblastoma cells.

Intermittent fasting makes weight loss and muscle building attainable. A majority of people who want to lose weight cannot stick to a diet. Fad diets turn into the latest craze but evaporate into thin air eventually. What's more, long-term use of any of these fad diets can result in serious deficits which yield detrimental effects to one's health. Some diets can result in water retention which can congest the heart; others result in water loss which can lead to dehydration, affecting the balance of sodium and potassium in the body; still, others which advocate an all-protein diet with no carbs can have dire consequences. Weight loss does occur, but has a pendulum or yo-yo effect on the health, the weight loss during the course of the diet is quickly gained back when the regimen is no longer in force. All this creates stress on the heart and organs, not to mention pressure on the part of the dieter to lose weight.

Another problem that many people face has to do with food restrictions. Without fail, these restrictions will become even more appealing and is often a cause for violations. For this reason, intermittent fasting presents a better option as a weight loss program. Some people maintain the notion that the hunger we feel is just a state of mind, and we need to communicate that idea to our bodies. Reality tells us that THIS IS DEFI-NITELY NOT SO! How would you console your hungry tummy, with all its musical growls that feeling hungry is just a state of mind? I cannot imagine how to tell a growling tummy to shut up!

Many people find the idea of fasting for twelve to 24 hours difficult since it involves behavior modification of deeply ingrained eating habits. At the start, there will surely be a transition period from "all the time eating" to "scheduled eating." The idea is to work it up gradually, from your normal eating pattern to an 8 to 10-hour window, then reduce it to 6 to 8 hours and even less if desired. Choose first whether you are going to skip breakfast or dinner and work around it accordingly. Know that it is okay to drink water, green or black tea or black coffee during your fasting period, but don't overdo it. There is no limit to the amount of pure water you can drink; and in fact, out of habit we typically reach for food or a snack when our bodies are actually crying for water instead.

Although difficulties will be encountered, it is the positive results that will be inspiring. Intermittent fasting is not just about overcoming the idea of hunger to be able to go without food for some time. It is more of establishing a new pattern of eating which can yield the desired benefits of weight loss and muscle shaping.

You will be surprised to discover that that **intermittent fasting can provide better mental clarity and concentration.** This is a great benefit of implementing the intermittent fasting pattern of eating be-cause it is important to have days filled with energy and mental clarity. This increases productivity and the creative output and puts you in an excellent mood for the day.

There are also many other benefits of intermittent fasting which involve the sympathetic and parasympathetic nervous system, but none of these benefits will be felt if you are only practicing fasting while sleeping. For best results a person with a highly active lifestyle should implement intermittent fasting for 16 hours; 24-hour fasts are recommended for those with a lower level of activity. This is what the "experts" say, but you don't have to make a drastic move just to find out that it doesn't work for you. I suggest that you make whatever transition slowly according to your own pace, but whatever you do, keep going.

Common Myths and Issues with Intermittent Fasting

Knowing human nature, we have to deal with our fears squarely, especially when it comes to lifestyle changes that veer away from the norms of family and society. Like most, we have been programmed to believe certain ideas to be true, because we have heard it being mouthed by people we respect. Some examples of these are:

Alcohol will fatten you up, so you may not take alcoholic drinks while fasting or on a diet. The truth is that the body has a hard time breaking down ethanol, let alone converting it to fat.

Short-term fasting decreases metabolic rate. Scientific studies show the exact opposite.

Breakfast is the most important meal of the day. The Kellogg Company has bombarded us with advertisements to this effect, so many of us believe that it's "breakfast first thing in the morning." We have heard the same statement from our grandparents and parents, and we could not leave for school without breakfast.

Cooked meals can be replaced by shakes, meal replacement powers, and protein bars. This is the answer to today's busy lifestyle, the coping mechanism of this get-up-and-go generation, but we know better. The oldies know that there is no substitute for sitting down to a nice warm meal.

But many have come to believe it because of

Repetition. We hear it being said over and over, and since many believe it, then it must be true.

Advertisements. We are constantly bombarded by TV commercials, print, and even pop-ups on our computer.

Knowledge deficit on the part of the general public. We need to educate ourselves, especially on things concerning our health.

There are eight notions (there could be more) which in one way or another may affect public acceptance of the intermittent fasting eating pattern, and these are

NOTION 1: **Fasting or dieting will ruin your metabolism and make you fat and hungry.**

ANSWER: There is a slight increase in metabolic rate in direct proportion to the number of calories consumed.

NOTION 2: **Eat smaller meals more often for hunger control**

ANSWER: It is not so much the frequency of the meal which will control hunger. If the meal is made up of carbohydrates and simple sugars, the body will burn these quickly and be hungry again in a short time. Moreover, if the body expects to be fed every few hours, there would be no motivation to seek other fuels to burn; add to that little or no activity, and the excess calories are stored as fat. Three high-protein balanced meals control appetite better than six high-protein meals. Aside from the change in composition, it would be wise to cut down on caloric density and increasing volume by replacing with cruciferous vegetables and complex carbohydrates.

NOTION 3: **Eat small meals regularly to keep blood sugar under control and provide an alert mind and energetic body.**

ANSWER: Blood sugar follows the meal pattern you are accustomed to. In normal individuals, blood sugar is naturally stable. In those with insulin resistance, stability is subject to the usual diet, food intake, hormone-regulated patterns, and hereditary factors.

There is no need to eat regularly to control blood sugar levels since blood sugar is able to maintain itself and adjusts to your chosen eating pattern,

NOTION 4: **Fasting switches the body gears into "starvation mode."**

ANSWER: After a meal, the body's metabolic rate increases and remains so until 60 hours after. There is no decrease in metabolic rate that occurs until after 60 hours of fasting. Therefore, to say that the body switches to "starvation mode" as a result of fasting is not true.

NOTION 5: **Consume proteins every 2-3**

hours to maintain a steady supply of amino acids.

ANSWER: This eating pattern would put the body under great stress. It takes more than 5 hours for the body to digest a standard meal, and amino acids are still being released into the blood and absorbed by muscles until much later. It all depends on the meal composition, such as a type of protein, carbohydrates, fiber and what was ingested during prior meals. These are the factors that determine how long amino acids will be made available to the tissues after meals. So after 5 hours, you are still "anabolic," essentially meaning that the energy from your food is still accessible for tissue growth and maintenance.

NOTION 6: **Fasting causes muscle loss.**

ANSWER: Just by changing meal frequency, the effect of regular fasting on muscle contour showed the fat loss and increased muscle gain even without changing calorie intake or weight training. The issue of catabolism does not become a problem with short-term controlled fasting. The body would not enter into a catabolic state, a condition that is mainly caused by excessive training in conjunction with inadequate protein nutrition unless there is impaired protein absorption coupled with long fasting periods daily. And this happens gradually when amino acids are not available from food, and stored liver glycogen is depleted.

NOTION 7: **Skipping breakfast is bad and will make you fat.**

ANSWER: Breakfast skippers are seen as those who engage in crash diets, have higher weight and BMI. After a fasting period through sleep, insulin sensitivity is highest in the morning, increased after glycogen depletion, and breakfast eater's exhibit better controls over their dietary habits. This is what made people think that breakfast is healthy and improves insulin sensitivity. Recent studies show otherwise.

NOTION 8: **Fasting increases cortisol.**

ANSWER: Cortisol increases in response to a stressor, to help the body's stress coping mechanism. This is related to the breakfast issue, in that breakfast eaters suffer post-breakfast hunger which is triggered by an in-crease in cortisol levels following an all-night fast; and misinterpreting these body signals triggers and all-day eating pattern. This increased cortisol level has benefits, which is why it was suggested to exercise early in the morning on an empty stomach because one can maintain an adequate rate of exertion for a long time without suffering pain, hunger, and fatigue. Cortisol increases wakefulness, alertness and memory recall. So used in conjunction with fasting, it has good effects. Bad effects will hap-pen if the exposure to a stressor is prolonged.

When we are accustomed to eating many times per day, the feeling of hunger in our body will normally cause panic, and we start looking for food. But, what happens if we don't get to consume that food? Absolutely nothing. Our health won't be threatened by missing a few meals.

There is a difference between psychological and physical hunger. When we feel hungry, the psychological hunger is present. We just think that we are hungry, but our body has enough fuel to function well. At this time, our body is burning the fat deposits, and we are slimming down. Some-times, eating is done out of habit and is a result of our thoughts. When we see a food commercial, we are psychologically stimulated to feel hunger, even if we have eaten an hour barely before.

By using intermittent fasting, we are putting our bodies and minds into a self-imposed rest period for a determined period of time. For some people, this period is simply the sleeping time. Interesting, right? If the last consumed meal is at eight pm, and the next time we eat is at eight am, there are twelve hours during which our body is fasting. Other people are deciding for some different type of fasting. For example, one meal is in the afternoon, and the next meal is consumed the next afternoon at the same time. You are probably wondering how this can be healthy and help you gain muscle. Well, it actually is. There have been many studies and experiments conducted on this subject that prove this is the healthiest way to lose surplus weight. The data collected by all of the research shows that with proper usage of intermittent fasting, people could extend the length of their life, regulate their blood pressure, regulate weight and easily gain lean muscle with exercise.

Simply put, intermittent fasting is not a magical formula which guarantees immediate results. It takes discipline and a conscious decision to follow through. But if you are new to intermittent fasting, take heart. If you decide that breakfast is the meal to skip, but on one of those days you feel like you need a break, go ahead and do it. Make your experience with intermittent fasting fun and exciting.

CHAPTER 3

TYPES OF INTERMITTENT FASTING

Several different methods can be tailored to individual needs and preferences. There are many familiar methods, but five of them are the most commonly used. It is not important which one is the most used or most desired by others, and it is important to find the method that works best for you and makes your life easier, which in turn make it easier to stick to this practice. Below is a brief overview of each of the five most commonly chosen methods for starting intermittent fasting.

The Daily Method, Also Known as Leangains

Initially introduced by Martin Berkhan, the Leangains method is a practice where fasting is performed for a 14 to 16 hour period and then allows a six to eight-hour window for eating. While the fasting period is on, you are not allowed to consume any calories. Of course, black coffee and sugar-free gum can be consumed, but it is better to stick to only pure water. For most people, this method is the best one because it allows them to enter into the routine easily and to see results faster. The period chosen for fasting can be during the night so that during some period of the day meals are allowed so that hunger won't discourage you so easily.

As mentioned before, fasting as a method can help to burn fat, but also to gain muscle instead of losing. To get the most from this method and get those sexy muscles, the kind of food you eat during the allowed feeding period is very important. It is well known that muscles are made in the kitchen, so let's see what is better to eat and when it is best to eat it. When working out, our body needs carbs to have the strength to with-stand the effort that exercising takes. The intake of protein should be on a high level, mostly every day depending on the gender, age, and fitness activity, in opposition to fats, which are allowed a higher intake only on the days when you are not exercising.

Martin Berkhan provides a few guidelines for those who are trying to gain muscle while practicing this method. According to him, on workout days there should be three meals eaten. If the first meal is close enough to the workout, it should include some carbs. The meal after the workout should be the largest meal eaten during the whole day, and you can include some dessert such as ice cream or maybe a piece of cheesecake. When you have a rest day, the calories consumed should be less than calories consumed on the workout day. On a rest day, the first meal should be your largest meal and should include a higher level of protein. There are also many other things to share, but these are the basics that will help you to get those lean muscles.

The Warrior Method

Introduced by Ori Hofmekler, the warrior diet is a fasting method that people who can follow the rules will be happy to put into practice. This diet works with twenty hours of fasting followed by one big meal. Eating a big meal is probably the key to this method. While the fasting period is on, you are able to have some fruit or vegetables, in low amounts of course. The permitted food intake is not at all a coincidence in this meth-od. Fresh food will increase the work of the nervous system by stimulating adrenaline that will contribute to fat burning. An interesting fact about this method is that the intake of food into the body only takes place during the nighttime hours, which subdues the nervous system and al-lows the spending of calories and improves the digestive process.

Another interesting thing is that this period provides relaxation and growth of muscles in the body. But, this can be misunderstood by some-one. Using this method, you should not expect to gain muscle as with the other methods, mainly because of the fact that food is limited to one meal during the night.

Of course, many people may find this way of losing weight pretty hard. Taking the main meal at night can be a serious problem for some people. Starvation throughout the day can also be a serious obstacle to overcome while practicing this method. But if someone has decided to practice it, they will endure throughout all of this.

Alternately Eating: Eat Stop Eat

Started by Brad Pilon, this method of fasting helps many people to lose weight and to boost their body. The concept behind this method is based on the following: you can eat everything you want during the week, except for one or two days when you shouldn't eat anything for 24 hours. As long as this period of fasting lasts, you can consume water, as well as some calorie-free drinks. The reason why some people find this method the perfect one for them is that they don't need to stay away from the things they want to eat; by fasting one or two days per week, they are lowering their calorie intake for the whole week, so they will manage to lose weight.

Even this method can be difficult for some people, but as its creator says, it is very efficient. It is a method that is flexible, and you can obtain the benefits of it as fast as you want. If you are not ready to put yourself in a fasting mode for whole 24 hours,

INTERMITTENT FASTING

you can start with as much time as you can manage to begin with and gradually increase the hours until you reach 24 hours. As with the first method, it is recommended to do some type of training, such as resistance training, so your body can burn fat and discover those lean, formed muscles much more quickly.

Fat Loss Forever Method

The fat loss forever method is an intermittent fasting method in cheating is allowed. This may be a great thing for people who like to lose weight but cannot stick to some strict diet or the hours of fasting that the other methods require. This method is actually a hybrid method created by Dan Go and John Romaniello, eliminating all the weaknesses that can be faced when practicing other methods. This program is often practiced for twelve weeks, in which one day per week you are allowed to cheat, and right after this day comes the 36 hours of fasting. This last number will scare most of us, right? The creators of this method suggest performing the fasting on the busiest days of the week, so we won't have a lot of time to think of food.

In addition to this method, there is a training program that can aid in gaining muscle and losing even more weight. Many people may find this method difficult, especially those who are not accustomed to fasting. The cheat days could be

221

threatening to some in the sense that during these days they could consume much more food than they normally would. But everything is in the self-control, isn't it?

Alternate Day Fasting

Alternate day fasting, also known as the Up Day, Down Day Diet, was created by James Johnson and is based on a simple philosophy. You should eat less for one day, and the next day you should eat as you normally do. This "less" means that during the fasting day, the calorie intake should be about 400 to 500 calories less than the days when you eat normally. For gaining muscle, exercising is recommended during the normal calorie days, since on low-calorie days you may find exercising difficult which could lead to discouragement.

This method is probably the easiest method to follow. But, what could happen with the usage of this method is that people may transform their normal calorie day into a lower calorie day, not noticing that it can cause them to challenge the results obtained with this way of fasting. Precisely for this reason, if this method is chosen, it is a good idea to plan in advance the meals for the next day in order to keep the level of calories within the desired frame.

Practicing intermittent fasting is a great way to learn how to control hunger and get in shape easy and fast. Using some of the methods mentioned above, you can easily stick to the fasting and maintain the fast for the de-sired length of time. The best thing that people can learn by practicing fasting is to control the hunger and recognize it for what it is. There are many examples that prove that this practice can lead to weight loss and building muscle.

CHAPTER 4

LOSING WEIGHT WITH INTERMITTENT FASTING

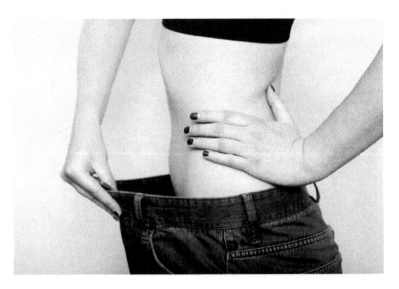

Weight loss is one of the most important reasons why people implement an intermittent fasting program in their lives. The weight loss benefits of this eating plan have been proven – in addition to assisting with metabolism, the diet also helps to curb your appetite, which means you will eat less.

With intermittent fasting, it is essential that you understand it is possible to gain weight instead of to lose weight if your diet is not appropriate. You will need to implement an appropriate diet in order to ensure that you achieve a caloric deficit, while still providing your body with the essential nutrients it relies on daily to perform all of the functions that are crucial to your own survival.

Different types of meal plans have been suggested for those people who are looking to lose weight through intermittent fasting. In the end, it is up to you to choose a meal plan that is appropriate for you. You will have to take yourself into account – consider how much weight you have to lose, and take into account any particular health conditions that you may be suffering from. These will all help you determine how many calories you should consume on a daily basis, how active you will need to be, and what types of food you will be able to include in your intermittent fasting diet plan.

The first step to losing weight with this type of eating habit would be to select an appropriate type of intermittent fasting program. We have al-ready discussed the various options out there that you can select from. Most people find that the standard 16/8 intermittent fasting program is ideal for them if they are only getting started. You can vary the number of days during the week that you will be following this program – some are also able to follow through with the 16/8 program for the entire week. You'll essentially have to listen to your own body – when you feel that you are starving yourself too much, adjust your plan in order to make up for the excessive reduction in your daily caloric consumption. On the other hand, if you find that you are not losing weight, it might be a good idea to take a look at your calorie balance – how much calories are you consuming and how much are you burning through physical activity?

Example Meal Plan for Weight Loss with Intermittent Fasting

If you do a quick search on Google for a weight loss plan that you can use with intermittent fasting, you will be surprised at just how many variations there are that you can choose from. This can really make the entire process challenging, instead of a fun and exciting journey that you are taking on in order to help you achieve a body that you will feel more confident about.

Many of the weight loss plans available can be effective if you stick to the plan and you ensure your body is provided with an adequate amount of exercise on a daily basis. Unfortunately, this does not make it easier to choose one that is ideal for yourself.

Below, we will take a look at an example of a really good intermittent fasting diet plan that you can follow and adjust according to your own preferences and requirements if you are finding it hard to choose an appropriate option for yourself. This is a very basic "framework" that you can work from.

Before we look at the example weight loss intermittent fasting meal plan – there is one thing that you should note. DO not expect everything to go smoothly the first time around. On your first few days, know that things can be rather difficult. This is especially true if you are used to eating continuously during the day – which is a very common problem among people who have a more significant amount of weight to lose.

Be patient in the beginning – with yourself and with the results you achieve through your diet plan. After a week or two, if you do not see the results that you expect, then aim to make a few adjustments in order to customize your diet plan and your intermittent fasting program to be more appropriate to your goals.

With the diet plan example that I am about to share with you – I want you to get into a habit of skipping breakfast. With the 16/8 program, you will only have a window between six to eight hours where you will consume food every day. Since you are aiming to lose weight, skipping out on breakfast means your body will start to utilize its own fat reserves in or-der to generate energy. This is ideal for someone who needs to lose weight.

You will have your first meal at 3 pm in the afternoon. Have your second meal at around 6 pm and then finish off the day with a final meal at around 10 pm.

Your first two meals of the day should be kept light. This way, you won't turn off your body's automatic fat burning mechanisms. By the end of the day, you'll consume a meal that is heavier on the calorie side. Even though you are free to experiment with the number of calories you consume during each meal, be wary of what food you decide to consume – you are trying to lose weight and become a healthier person. For this rea-son, always ensure that you eat healthily as well.

I personally recommend that the first two meals of your day should be a maximum of 400 calories each. Be sure that there is an adequate supply of protein in these meals. Don't skim on vegetables and fruits – enjoy them as they are good for you.

Here are some examples of small and light meals that you may wish to experiment with for your first two meals (at 3 pm and at 6 pm):

- Add some almonds and a couple of berries into a cup of Greek yogurt.
- Have some cottage cheese with a couple of almonds.
- Add one tablespoon of olive oil to a can of tuna, and enjoy your meal with an apple.
- Use two whole eggs to make yourself an omelet. Have this meal with some delicious berries.

If you are in the mood for a meatier meal, then cook up a chicken breast and enjoy it with a green salad. You can add half of an Avocado to the meal, as well as an apple.

For those who are in a hurry and would like to drink something instead, mixing a cup of unsweetened almond milk with about 40 grams of whey protein powder is a really good option. You can have some fruit with this, as well as about 20 grams of almonds.

When it comes to the third meal of the day – this is when you should enter the kitchen and prepare something healthy and delicious-tasting for yourself. There are a lot of different healthy meals that you can choose to fill the gap at 10 pm. It is a good idea to limit the last meal of the day to around 800 calories, but you can push it up to around 1000 calories if you wish.

When it comes to your last meal, it is important to balance fats and protein perfectly to avoid weight gain or other potential side-effects from your diet plan. If you are opting for a leaned piece of meat (to supply your body with quality protein), then you can have more healthy types of fats in your meal. If, on the other hand, you decide to opt for a fattier type of meal, let's say a piece of beef steak that is a fatty cut, then you should limit how much-added fats you put into your meal.

To help you prepare your third and final meal of the day, here are three examples of meals that are nutritious and will give you that final amount of calories that you need during your eating window:

• Cook up a chicken breast and serve it with some

potato wedges and a variety of vegetables.

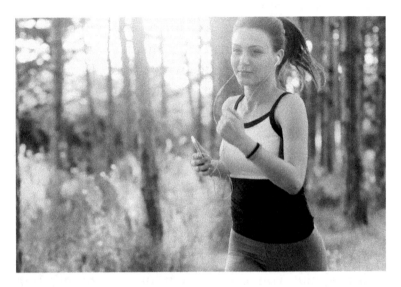

- Serve some brown rice with vegetables and a chicken breast. Try to use a small amount of coconut oil to cook both the rice and the chicken.
- If you are rather in the mood for some beef, then have a steak with some vegetables. You can also serve this up with a sweet potato – add a little bit of cinnamon to the sweet potato for additional flavor.

Exercising with Intermittent Fasting

Ask anyone who had successful results with any type of dieting program in the past – and they would tell you that exercise was a crucial part of their weight loss program. The primary idea behind any type of diet that aims to help you reduce your body weight is to create a caloric deficit. A caloric deficit simply means the number of calories you burn each day through your exercise protocols are higher than the number of calories you consume, as we have already discussed.

Thus, when you are implementing a diet plan along with intermittent fasting to help you lose weight, then you should ensure that you also implement an appropriate exercise program.

Some people are concerned about exercising while following a program that utilizes intermittent fasting strategies. However, once your body is used to this new eating style, you'll notice that it becomes easier and easier. There are also a variety of supplements that you can take to boost your endurance and stamina and to give you that extra energy that you will need to ensure you can get past a training session, even while you are fasting.

Here's a little-known secret that many people do not realize in terms of exercising while you are on an intermittent fasting program: the fat burning mechanisms of the human body is regulated by what is known as the sympathetic nervous system. This system is also called the SNS for short. When the system activates, it means your body starts to burn fat. There are two essential elements that cause the SNS system to activate – this includes a lack of food in your body, as well as exercise. When you decide to give your body a dose of both, then activation is more thorough, and your SNS will lead to a much more significant level of fat burning and weight loss.

There are many other benefits that should be

taken into account in terms of exercising while you are fasting. One particular benefit that becomes especially useful for those people who are trying to bulk up with muscle mass while they are following a plan that uses intermittent fasting is the fact that exercising during your fast window will cause oxidative stress. While oxidative stress is often considered a bad thing for the body, during exercise, it can actually be good for improving your muscle strength and mass.

Take this into account as well – if you eat before you participate in an exercise program, then there is a chance that the food you consumed may lead to issues with your general performance during your routine. It has been found that the consumption of food in any form – be it a shake, an energy bar, or an actual meal – causes your blood glucose levels to experience a spike while you are exercising. Sure, this will give you some energy to kickstart that tough routine that you are about to start – but, once this spike is over, your blood glucose levels will quickly decline, and you will basically experience a "crash." What this means is you will feel the fatigue coming on quickly, leading to poor muscle performance and a body that is quickly running out of energy.

There are, however, some publications that say this is a myth – but this is still something that you should consider when it comes to intermittent fasting!

All-in-all, there is a specific number of benefits that you may expect from a good workout program integrated into your intermittent fasting plan. You will be able to experience the following potential benefits with this particular combination:

- You can turn back what is known as the "biological clock" on your brain, as well as your muscles, due to the effects of exercise on your body while in a fasting state.
- The concentration of growth hormone produced by your body will be increased.
- Your body composition will be greatly improved, as you will experience a reduction in body fat percentage, along with an increase in lean muscle mass.
- Cognitive function will also benefit, and you'll find that problems like brain fog start to disappear.
- Your testosterone levels are likely to rise as well, which can be especially beneficial for older men who are experiencing a natural de-cline in the level of circulating testosterone within their bodies.

While exercising while fasting is definitely beneficial for you and your weight, there is one particular factor that I have to mention here. On days when you are going to do some heavy lifting as part of your exercise routine, it is crucial that you get your timing right. When you decide to participate in some heavy lifting exercises, then you will need to ensure you eat something within the first 30 minutes after you have completed the heavy lifting workout.

CHAPTER 5

CAN YOU BUILD LEAN MUSCLE WITH INTERMITTENT FASTING?

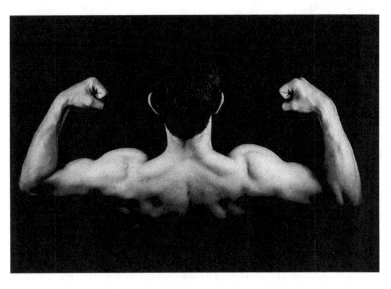

Practicing intermittent fasting has a proven impact on reducing body weight. Of course, the practice of exercising is an additional way to re-duce weight and is important not only when fasting, but always because it helps us to protect and maintain our general health. When following a fasting method, it is better to stick to some type of plan which can pro-vide even better results. Many are reluctant to accept this way of eating, when their main purpose is to create muscle, knowing that in the world of fitness getting a muscular body requires a very different diet. Fasting might seem daunting to many knowing that you should not eat for a period of approximately 16 hours of daylight, depending on the method chosen to be practiced. But when you consider that we spcnd eight hours in bed, and you go by the rule of no eating at least two hours before going to bed, you can easily endure an additional five to eight hours of fasting.

Below are some guidelines that can help you get the best results from intermittent fasting.

When fasting, try low-intensity cardio. When fasting, our body receives fewer calories during that meal than what is allowed. With fewer received calories, high-intensity cardio exercises can cause the opposite effect. Our body will show us what intensity is sufficient, beginning to experience shortness of breath is a sign that we need to stick to that intensity.

Try to exercise a few hours after you've eaten. After you consume a meal, the body begins to break down fats, sugars, carbohydrates, etc. In return, the body releases glycogen which acts as fuel for the body during exercise. At the same time, this way removes the risk of lowering blood sugar which will make us feel weak and exhausted if its levels become too low.

The entry of large amounts of protein will put you closer to your goal. To be able to put into practice the intermittent fasting and also build a strong and well-muscled body during the time in which eating is allowed, you need to consume greater amounts of protein. The exact timing of the intake of proteins which, along with carbohydrates, should be a few hours before exercise as well as after the completion of the exercise, will help make it easier to complete the training and build the de-sired muscle.

It is good to include snacks throughout the day. If the method you selected for fasting time allows, the intake of snacks during certain time periods will help blood sugar levels to remain normal. By maintaining normal blood sugar levels, we can have the energy to be able to practice the exercises properly and do more repetitions which will contribute to the combustion of a large quantity of fat.

Although perhaps this practice will run into some of the mistrust, if the food is consumed properly, the muscles can be easily built. The first thing that should be done for successful implementation of occasional fasting in the process of building muscle is to determine the level of required calories for your body. This course is individual and different for every person. After you determine the required amount of calories, you need to decide on a pre-workout to take around twenty percent of total daily calories. This dish should be eaten just before the workout and need to contain sufficient carbs which will certainly give energy and proteins which are essential for muscle growth. The rest of the required daily calories should be distributed through the rest of the time after a workout while fasting has not started. This may involve a lot of food for many, especially if training is late in the afternoon, but with the right choice of food, calories will certainly help. The way the occasional fasting helps in terms of building muscle is that after the training the body needs carbo-hydrates to help regain strength; the intake of large amounts of fat can be harmful in these moments. Precisely for this reason, you can choose a larger meal containing carbs and protein, which allows the combination of fat and protein to remain for several hours after training, in order to reduce the need for carbohydrates in large quantities.

Stay hydrated

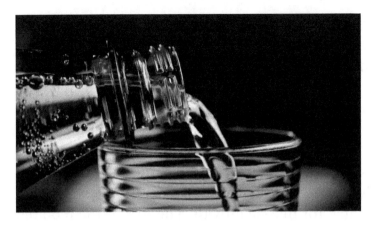

We all are aware that 95% of our body is made up of water. The introduction of a certain amount of water, from 1.5L to 3L depending on the individual, is important not only for the occasional practice of fasting but al-so for maintaining health in everyday life. But the reason I mention this is not just that. It is because with the consumption of water, we suppress hunger and it is easier to deal with methods that are designed for fasting.

Water is important for balancing the body's different systems such as the heart, brain, kidneys, lungs and of course, the biggest one, muscles. On the other hand, the intake of the required amount of water is important because the muscles need water for moisture and growth. Water is also important because we flex and move our muscles. If we do not drink enough water during the day, our body will become dehydrated, and muscle control and strength will be impaired. With the proper amount of water, we can easily build strong muscles and get the best results from the training. Dehydration will also lead to unhealthy, sagging skin and slower muscle response.

Measure the results and stay motivated

Seeing results always give the greatest motivation. In terms of weight loss, it can often be disappointing if we do not begin to see the results of our efforts quickly. That is the reason why many people try to reduce excess weight before starting. The practice of occasional fasting gives visible results in a short period of time if properly practiced.

The results that occasionally gives can be quite impressive. With proper usage of certain exercises, (depending on the purpose of the current training, or whether our goal is to create a lithe body with lean muscles or a body with large, defined muscles) muscles will gradually increase, pushing out the fat, until they become visible. What must be noted is that you should not rely on scales, for the simple reason that weight is increased due to the building of muscle, which weighs more than fat. The best way to monitor results is with images. Before the occasional fasting combined with the training that you alone will determine, take a picture of yourself and remember the date. Each subsequent week or month, take a new photograph, and you will be amazed when you see how your body is changing. Each week your muscle will be hidden by less fat deposits.

CHAPTER 6

DEVELOPING AN INTERMITTENT FASTING MEAL PLAN

Once you have decided to start with an intermittent fasting program – whether it is to help you lose weight and get healthier or to take advantage of other health benefits that have been associated with this eating style – you will need to go through a phase where you will plan for the big change that is coming up. You'll have to choose the type of intermit-tent fasting plan you would like to follow, and you need to decide how you will be implementing this type of eating plan into your own life.

It is important to not just jump into intermittent fasting without planning out how you will go about your new diet plan first. Without a solid plan, you might end up cheating, eating the wrong foods, or doing things in such a wrong way that you may experience serious side effects from your new diet.

One of the most important things that you need to target when you are planning out your intermittent fasting program would be the meal plan. Most people find that it is much easier to continue following an intermit-tent fasting program if they know what they will have for dinner or what snacks they should pack for when that time comes when they can start catching up on the time they spent committed to fasting.

For some people, it can be difficult to set up a meal plan that will be effective. It is essential, as described already, to ensure a meal plan fits in with the specific goals that you might be striving for with intermittent fasting.

Before you can start to plan out your meals while you are going to be following an intermittent fasting program, make sure that you know exactly what your goals are and why are you planning to implement this pro-gram. Do you want to lose weight? Would you like to build muscle at the same time? Are you simply looking to try out intermittent fasting for other types of benefits? Your goals will ultimately help you set up a meal plan that will allow you to reach them and to take advantage of what intermittent fasting is able to offer you.

In addition to considering the goals that you are striving toward with intermittent fasting, you will also need to take into account the type of intermittent fasting program that you will be following. Some allow you to eat for specified times during the day, and others require fasting for the major part of the day. There are different options available – and we have already looked at the options that you can choose from.

Since there are so many varieties of intermittent fasting to choose from, we would really need a completely separate book to look at every type of meal plan that you could develop in order to set up an appropriate plan for your journey. To make things simpler, we will take a look at one or two examples of meal plans that you could follow. This will give you an idea of what to expect, what type of foods to include, and more.

Examples of Meal Plans for 16/8 Intermittent Fasting Option

Example #1

Let's start by taking a look at a meal plan for the 16/8 intermittent fasting model. With this particular option, you would fast for 16 hours of the day and then enjoy eight hours where you are allowed to eat. The following is just a simple example of a meal plan – you can take from it and make appropriate modifications in order to include the foods that you require to achieve your goal.

You would start the day with a fresh cup of black coffee – no milk or creamer, and absolutely no sugar. This will help to give your digestive system and metabolism a good kickstart for the day, without adding calories to your day.

Coffee has a host of benefits for your body, which is why it is a great idea to get your day off with a good cup of coffee. You can choose your favorite blend – the most important part here is that you enjoy your coffee with no sugar or milk.

After you had your coffee, get your day started. Try to keep yourself active. If you keep busy, you're less likely to think about eating something. You'll keep your mind distracted and yourself on track with your intermittent fasting diet plan. During this time, you should ensure that you drink an adequate amount of water.

As the day goes by, you should try to stay strong. By around 3 pm, if you do feel the hunger coming on, try to drink a sparkling water drink. Aim for one that does not contain any calories. There are various flavored sparkling waters on the market that are available in zero-calorie options. The sparkling water will usually help to make your stomach feel at least a little fuller and can be a great tool for getting yourself through that final push until you can have something to eat.

When the time comes to break your fasting period and start to enjoy food, try to do it slowly. Avoid pushing a 500-gram steak down your throat. Start with something simple, such as a protein bar. There are protein bars that are packed with useful nutrients, along with a high amount of protein, but still low on the calorie part. Consider this a treat – a way to reward yourself for keeping strong and pushing through the entire fasting period.

Wait about an hour and then have a fruit. An apple is a really great choice in this case. Apples are extremely nutritious, and they taste great – plus they contain a lot of water and apples are low in calories. You can cut the apple into small slices and then enjoy them slice-by-slice. In addition to tasting great, the apple will also give you a burst of energy that should help you get through the period until you are going to have dinner.

If you do feel the need to have another snack before dinner time strikes, try to have some water first. If you feel hungry after the water, then try to aim for a low-calorie snack. Limit yourself to about 100 calories – but only have a snack if it is absolutely necessary. Perhaps have another fruit.

Try to prepare dinner so that you can enjoy it at around 6.30pm to 7.00pm. Dinner can be big, but should still consist of healthy food choices. There is no use in trying to take advantage of the benefits that intermittent fasting has for your well-being when you are just going to smack a McDonald's burger down your throat the moment you get a chance to eat.

Perhaps prepare some brown rice with chicken, or maybe some home-made meatballs with spaghetti. Try to include some vegetables as well. There is no need to limit yourself to just one or two different meals. There are thousands of recipes all over the internet that you can enjoy – just be sure that there are not too many calories in the meal and ensure the ingredients are good for you.

Before you go to bed, aim to get a few more calories into your body. At around 10 pm, you can treat yourself with a little snack. Aim for some-thing that is below around 400 calories to avoid stuffing your body with a lot of calories just before you go to sleep. A good idea at this time would be a bar or a cookie, or anything else that contains a high amount of protein.

Example #2

Let's take a look at another example of how you can use the intermittent fasting program to help you reach your specific goals. In this example, we are going to consider those who are only starting out with intermittent fasting and still find that it is incredibly difficult to make the adjustment that is needed. Thus, the fasting window will only last for 14 hours per day, instead of 16, and the eating window is extended to 10 hours, instead of only eight hours.

Planning Your Meals for Specific Goals

The example meal plan discussed above is a good option if you are trying to lose weight, but not all people who are opting for an intermittent fasting diet will want to lose weight. At the beginning of this book, we dis-cussed the various benefits that this type of eating plan could have – so there are other reasons why people are choosing to follow an intermit-tent fasting diet as well.

You will need to take such factors into account.

For example, let's say you want to bulk up and gain some lean muscle mass while you are following a diet that takes advantage of intermittent fasting – you will need to aim at increasing your intake of calories through the periods in which you are allowed to eat. This can be quite difficult since the window can be somewhat small.

If you go about this all in a smart way, then you will be able to achieve an ideal number of calories during the day, and you will gain enough protein and other nutrients to support your body, as well as reach your goal of bulking up.

There are many high-protein foods that you can include in your diet and consume them throughout your eating window. Try out some Greek yogurt, or perhaps cook up some cheese quesadilla. A single serving of cheese quesadilla contains around 10 grams worth of protein. A serving of Greek yogurt can offer you about 13 grams of protein. There are many different options – try to be creative and find ways to integrate these protein-rich foods into your meal plan.

Calculating Your Daily Macro Requirements

When it comes to following a diet, it is always useful to <u>calculate your specific daily macro requirements</u> in order to know how much food you should consume, and the specific types of food you should ideally consume. There are three macros that you will need to focus on – this includes proteins, fats, and, of course, carbohydrates.

In most cases, whether you are trying to recompose your body, lose weight, or gain muscle mass, you will focus on achieving a relatively high protein intake. On some days, your fat intake will be lower than others. Carbohydrate intake should always make up for the remaining calories that are left after you have determined the amount of protein and fat to consume in your daily diet.

You will generally also have different macro requirements for days when you will be training, compared to those days where you will not be training and will rather take a resting day instead.

Determine Your Daily Caloric Intake Requirement.

Before we can discuss how your daily macro requirements can be calculated, we first need to look at how you can determine the most ideal number of calories that you should consume each day.

There are different strategies that can be used to help you determine your ideal daily caloric requirements. Below, we will use a basic system known as the "Harris-Benedict formula" to help you determine the best number of calories that you should consume. I will lay this out in a step-by-step manner to make things easier for you:

1.   The first step is to calculate your BMR. This is a figure that is generally considered the number of calories that your body will re-quire to survive

if you are physically inactive – particularly when you might be in a coma. This really is a two step process, so follow both of the steps I outline below:

- a. Calculate your Lean Body Mass with the following formula -> LBM = weight – (weight * (body fat percentage / 100)).
- b. Calculate your BMR with the following formula -> BMR = 370 + 21.6 * LBM (Note: LBM / Lean Body Mass should be in kilograms)

2. Next, you will need to make a couple of adjustments to your BMR. Start by considering your physical activity level. The more physically active you are, the more you will need to eat on a day-to-day basis. Follow the following formulas to calculate your TDEE.

- a. If you do not exercise much and live a sedentary lifestyle, then the formula is 1.2 x BMR
- b. If you participate in light activities up to three times per week, then the formula is 1.375 x BMR
- c. If you are moderately active and participate in physical activity up to five days per week, then the formula is 1.55 x BMR
- d. If you are very active and take part in training programs or sports for seven days per week, then the formula is 1.725 x BMR
- e. If you are extremely active and participate in heavy workouts multiple times each day,

then the formula is 1.9 x BMR

3.   Once you have calculated your TDEE, the next part of the process is to consider your specific goals. There are three particularly popular goals that people often strive toward when they consider implementing intermittent fasting. This includes fat loss, muscle gain, and body recomposition. The specific goal that you are striving to will have an impact on how you should adjust your daily caloric consumption as follow:

a.   If you want to gain muscle mass, then add 20% to the TDEE you calculated previously.

b.   If you want to lose weight, then you need to consider your current body fat percentage. Follow this guide to understand how much you should reduce your caloric intake in order to achieve your goal:

i.   Body fat percentage of 30% or higher -> reduce daily calorie intake by 30%

ii.   Body fat percentage between 20% and 30% -> reduce daily calorie intake by 25%

iii.   Body fat percentage between 10% and 20% -> re-duce daily calorie intake by 20%

iv.   Body fat percentage under 10% -> reduce daily calorie intake by 15%

c.   If you want to recomposition your body, then do not make any adjustments to your daily caloric intake.

Now that you have an idea of the average daily caloric intake you should achieve to reach your goals through intermittent fasting, there is an important step left – caloric intake should defer on training days and resting days.

It is generally recommended to have a 40% different between these days.

• On your resting days, you should follow this formula to determine how many calories you should consume: calculated daily calorie in-take x 0.8

• On training days where you will participate in physical activities, follow this formula: calculated daily calorie intake x 1.2

Calculating Your Ideal Macros

Now that you know how many calories you need to consume on specific days of the week, the next step would be to calculate the ideal amount of each macro that should make up your diet.

I usually start by setting my own protein intake level – protein should be kept high as it is the building block for your muscles. In addition to protein's effect on muscles, this is also a satiating macro, which means you'll feel fuller when the majority of your meal consists of protein.

It is generally recommended to calculate your protein intake based on your lean body mass, with a recommendation between 2.3 and 3.1 grams of protein per one kilogram of body weight. For me, the ideal amount is 2.5 grams of protein per kilogram body weight, but each person is different.

If this amount does not work for you, then adjust your protein intake accordingly.

Fat intake is usually also calculated based on your lean body mass. The recommended range is between 0.9 and 1.3 grams of fat per one kilogram of body weight. Make sure that you gain fat from healthy sources and not from takeaway French fries!

When you deduct the number of calories in the fat and protein sources that you will be consuming, the remainder should be filled with carbohydrates. Each one gram of carbohydrates will give you a total of four calories.

CHAPTER 7

TIPS FOR GETTING STARTED WITH INTERMITTENT FASTING

Most people who are used to their daily routine of having three meals and never skipping out will find it intimidating to get started with implementing intermittent fasting into their lives. This especially goes for those individuals who eat multiple times a day and who have a particularly hard time controlling their cravings. With intermittent fasting, it is vital that you stick to your schedule for maximum benefits. That said, there is no need to act like you are in a military camp.

With some simple steps, you can make the entire process of adopting intermittent fasting a fun journey for yourself – an experimental procedure that will take some time to perfect, but once you get there, you will be able to master this technique and gain many health benefits. Keep this in mind when you feel like quitting – you will only be able to reach that goal if you keep yourself motivated at all times.

Before you jump into intermittent fasting, you might want to take some things into consideration first. In particular, if you have been diagnosed with any type of chronic disease and if you are taking medications, then you should first talk with your physician to determine if this is a safe option for you.

Furthermore, don't overcomplicate things. Start small. Break the process up into small steps. Reach for smaller goals and ultimately aim for that big goal of fully implementing fasting techniques into your life. If you cave or something goes wrong, do not let it get you down. Instead, just keep on going.

Here Is a Step-By-Step Guide to Help You Out.

The first step is to determine what type of technique you want to adopt. The 16/8 is highly recommended for beginners. What you may not know is that you are already halfway there. You are fasting while you are sleeping – we bet you haven't thought of this before… Now, to get to the 16/8, you will simply have to start skipping breakfast, for example.

Decide on the time slots – dedicate eating windows and fasting windows. If you follow the 16/8 plan, for example, you can decide to have your first meal of the day at lunchtime, instead of early in the morning, and finish off at 8 PM, for example. Give yourself a good 16 hours without food – this would include your seven to nine hours of sleep, which you should be getting to keep your body healthy.

Start small and simple – try this for one day and see if you can make it. If you feel like you run out of energy too quickly, then stretch your eating window a little and make your fasting window narrower. As the days go by, start to shorten your eating window and make your fasting window longer – that is until you can go without food for 16 hours at a time. If you make a mistake by giving in to the temptation of having a snack when the hunger becomes extreme, don't beat yourself up over it. Simply start over.

In addition to deciding on the perfect option for you, it is also a good idea to consider why you want to include intermittent fasting in your life. When you are doing this for a specific purpose, then you will have some-thing to keep you motivated. Perhaps you want to lose weight. This is a great reason to fast – remember we looked at scientific evidence before that supported the weight loss advantages of intermittent fasting...

If you want simply want to help prolong your lifespan and reduce your risk of certain diseases, then these are also important reasons. Write them down if you have to – on your schedule. This will keep you motivated to ensure you can reach your goal.

Apps and Tools That Will Make Your Journey

Easier

Things can become confusing, especially at first, when you start with intermittent fasting. This is why using some essential tools to help you keep track of everything would be a good idea. You can always go old school and decide to plot down your schedule on a piece of paper. Perhaps buy a new notebook that is dedicated to this journey you are about to go on. Write down your schedule and mark down your progress. This will also help you go back and track your performance, as well as see where you have slipped up – giving you the ability to identify opportunities for improvement in the future.

If you rather prefer to keep things digital, then try out a couple of intermittent fasting apps. You would be surprised at how many there are. Take a look at some – they are available on both Google Play Store and Apple Store. Consider the user reviews. Then decide on an app that you like – and try to use it every day to help you keep track of your journey.

LIFE is currently one of the top-rated apps used for this purpose. It gives you the ability to record data for any type of intermittent fasting method that you would like to follow. You can easily adjust your schedule, and the app will even tell you when your body is expected to be in the ketosis phase. To keep you inspired and motivated, the app also allows you to join groups of other people who are on the same journey as you are.

CHAPTER 8

WHO SHOULD AVOID INTERMITTENT FASTING?

While intermittent fasting is generally considered a safe and effective lifestyle decision and a way of eating, there are some cases where this particular diet may not be the most appropriate option for a person. It is important that individuals who are interested in adopting an intermittent fasting diet first consider the pros and cons of this diet, and take a look at the specific risks that have been associated with this way of eating. If the individual finds that they might fall within the risky side of things, then intermittent fasting may not be an ideal option for them. In such cases, the person may be better off opting for an alternative diet that can help them achieve their specific goals.

As with any type of meal plan and adjustment to

how you are eating, it can be beneficial to first consult with a physician on intermittent fasting before you start to implement such a plan into your own life. It is best to choose a physician that already knows you and your medical history – this way, and the physician will be able to determine if you would be a good candidate for intermittent fasting and if a different type of diet might be more appropriate for you.

Women should especially ensure they consult with their physician before they decide to start following an intermittent fasting diet. The reason for this is because intermittent fasting has been found to have an adverse impact on the hormonal balance within a woman's body in some cases. When a woman's hormones are not in balance, then she may experience a number of potential adverse effects.

Some potential adverse events that a woman may experience when her hormones are out of balance may include:

• Developing skin-related problems. Dry skin is quite common amongst women who have an imbalance in hormones within their body. Another very common issue that this particular problem may cause is the development of pimples. Skin discolorations may also occur in some cases. These can all cause a woman to experience problems in terms of their mental health – they may start to feel self-conscious about their appearance.

• Brain fog may also develop when a woman's

hormones are out of balance. This can be an extremely dreadful issue, as the woman may find that they are unable to focus and concentrate, and their memory may also be adversely affected. In turn, the woman will experience a significant decline in their productivity. With this in mind, their time at work will be less effective.

• In addition to brain fog, many women find that they develop fatigue – often quite frequently – with an imbalance in their hormone levels. Fatigue can be just as dreadful. The woman may find that she feels tired all the time and wants to sleep a lot.

• Mood swings are also relatively common among women with issues in terms of their hormonal balance. Along with the mood swings may come sessions of anxiety and stress, as well as depression.

• In some cases, a woman may also find that their libido becomes low with inadequate regulation of their hormones. With a low libido, the woman will not be interested in participating in sexual intercourse with their partner.

People who are suffering from certain conditions will also need to be careful when it comes to implementing an intermittent fasting plan into their life. Some of the conditions that are considered risk factors for experiencing adverse effects when it comes to intermittent fasting include adrenal fatigue, existing hormonal issues, and gastrointestinal problems. Furthermore, people who have a history of eating disorders are also ad-vised to avoid intermittent fasting as this may yield unpleasant results potentially.

CHAPTER 9

THE SCIENTIFIC EVIDENCE BEHIND INTERMITTENT FASTING

When it comes to learning more about specific types of diet plans and lifestyle habits, it is always important to take a look at the scientific re-search behind such programs. With this in mind, the same applies to those who are interested in taking on an intermittent fasting plan – whether it is to lose weight or to build muscle mass or to enjoy a healthy way of living simply and to experience the benefits. If you are interested in intermittent fasting, be sure to first take a good look at the scientific evidence behind this eating plan. Do not only consider the potential benefits that intermittent fasting might have for you, but also consider the possible side-effects and downsides that may apply to those who are following a diet that is based on intermittent fasting.

Many scientific studies have been done on intermittent fasting, which can help you determine the efficiency and safety of this particular diet program. In this chapter, I would like to go over a few of the previous studies that have been conducted.

"Daily fasting works for weight loss, finds the report on 16:8 diet."
https://www.sciencedaily.com/releases/2018/06/180618113038.htm

The University of Illinois at Chicago published the results of a recent study they conduct, titled Daily fasting works for weight loss, finds the report on 16:8 diet. The study was officially published on ScienceDaily on the 18th of June, 2018.

The study focused on obtaining data relevant to the effects of intermit-tent fasting on the body weight of individuals who are obese. There was a total of 23 volunteers who participated in the study. All of the volunteers were obese, with a BMI that measured 35 or higher. The average age of the participants was about 45.

During the study, the participants were asked to consume their meals be-tween 10 am in the morning and 6 pm at night During the rest of the day, the participant was asked to undergo a fast – where they were not al-lowed to consume any type of food or beverages, except for water and selected beverages that do not contain calories. This particular study lasted for a total of 12 weeks.

Several benefits were noted by the scientists who were involved in the study. The results that were obtained in this study were compared to results from a previous study that also focused on the effects of fasting on obesity and body weight, but that previous study did not implement time-restricted fasting protocols.

In particular, this study found that weight loss was much more significant among those individuals who followed an intermittent fasting diet plan. Calorie consumption was also reduced by a statistically significant level. In addition to the weight-related benefits, it was also found that the study participants experienced an improvement in their blood pressure levels. With obesity being linked to high blood pressure – and this condition, in turn, associated with a range of adverse effects in the body, including blood vessel damage, this is certainly a benefit that needs to be noted.

The average participant in this particular study was found to consume 350 calories less than they did before they started to follow the intermit-tent fasting diet that was presented to them by the researchers involved in the study. Additionally, the individuals involved in the study were also found to lose an average of 3% of their total body weight. Additionally, systolic blood pressure levels were decreased by an average of seven millimeters per mercury, or mm Hg.

Scientists involved in the study concluded by saying that the obese population should know that there are ways that they can lose weight effectively without the need for excessively starving themselves, without having to count calories to the last digit, and without the need to eliminate all of the most tasteful foods that they are used to consuming.

It should be noted that results in this particular study on intermittent fasting and the diet's effect on weight loss had similar results compared to the previous studies that focused on fasting in general in terms of insulin resistance, cholesterol regulation, and fat mass. Still, this holds important evidence that intermittent fasting can be a good tool in a person's weight loss strategy.

"Intermittent fasting interventions for the treatment of overweight and obesity in adults."

A study conducted scientists at the University of Glasgow in the United Kingdom, published on the 1st of February 2018, looked at how intermit-tent fasting could be utilized as an intervention in the treatment of excessive weight among adults in the local region. The study was conducted in such a way to compare the results obtained with intermittent fasting to the results that can be achieved through no treatment, as well as through more traditional means of treating obesity in adult patients.

All of the patients who were part of the study had a BMI that was more than 25, which classifies them as being overweight. A large number of the study participants were obese as well, which means their BMI was higher than 30. All of the participants were over the age of 18 at the time of the study.

Each patient who participated in the study were provided with a diet plan that they had to follow. On intermittent fasting days, the patient was ad-vised to consume a diet that resulted in less than 800 kcal in total consumption per day. The study lasted for 12 weeks in total to ensure adequate time for results to be achieved, as it is known that appropriate weight loss results with any changes in diet can take a while.

The most significant results noted by this study were the reduction in the body weight of the participants who were involved in the intermittent fasting diet. In addition to these primary outcomes of the study, there were several secondary outcomes that the scientists who were involved in the study noted as well.

The secondary outcomes presented by the study was divided into multiple groups, and consists of:

- Anthropometric outcomes: Participants had a lower BMI at the end of the study and smaller waist circumference. Fat mass and fat-free mass were also reduced significantly, compared to the other studies that were compared to the results obtained from the intermittent fasting programs.

- Cardio-metabolic outcomes: Blood glucose levels were improved, along with insulin levels. The study also noted statistically significant improvements in the blood pressure levels of patients who participated in the intermittent fasting program. Lipoprotein pro-files had also improved.

It should be noted that some results obtained in

the intermittent fasting study were very similar to the results that were obtained in the other studies that these results were compared to.

In the end, this is yet another study that provides evidence of the effective results that intermittent fasting can provide a person with if they follow through on the particular plan that has been developed for them. Dedication and patience are two key factors to ensure the individual following this type of diet is able to achieve success and reach the goals they have set out for themselves.

"Intermittent Fasting with or without Exercise Prevents Weight Gain and Improves Lipids in Diet-Induced Obese Mice" *https://www.ncbi.nlm.nih.gov/pmc/articles/PMC5872764/*

While many people tend to exclude animal-based studies when they are looking for evidence on a specific topic, it is important to consider the fact that these animal-studies pave an important way for future human studies to be implemented. Thus, I would like us to take a look at one particular study in the MDPI Nutrients Journal, published on the 12th of March 2018. The study looked at how intermittent fasting would affect the potential of gaining weight, as well as the lipid profiles, in mice that were purposely made obese through a specific diet that they were fed.

In this study, laboratory rats were fed a diet that

was high in sugar and fat for 24 weeks in total. The diet was induced upon them at the age of eight weeks. After the 24-week period had concluded, the mice were divided into five appropriate groups in order to gain a more accurate insight into how beneficial intermittent fasting would be for weight loss, the prevention of weight gain, and more.

These five groups consisted of the following:

- Baseline control
- No intervention
- Intermittent Fasting
- High-intensity interval training, or HIIT
- Combination group, which included both high-intensity interval training and intermittent fasting protocols.

Several factors were taken into account during this study. The body com-position and general strength of each mouse were analyzed, along with a number of blood variables. Measurements were taken before the study was officially started, as well as at week 10 and at week 12.

The groups that had intermittent fasting included in their program all experienced a significant reduction in weight gain, even when fed a diet that induced obesity. Fat accumulation in these groups was also much lower than in the groups that did not include intermittent fasting. In addition to these benefits, the scientists that were in charge of the study al-so noted that the lipoprotein levels in the laboratory rats (in particular, their LDL cholesterol) were reduced significantly as well.

These results were observed in the group of mice that were simply placed on an intermittent fasting program, as well as those who had an intermit-tent fasting program along with high-intensity interval training.

The conclusion of the study was that intermittent fasting could result in assistance to reduce the risk of excess weight gain. The diet can also be useful for reducing fat accumulation in the body and may also be useful for improving cholesterol balance. These results can be achieved even when intermittent fasting is implemented without an active exercise plan, according to the evidence presented by this study.

Further research is still needed among human subjects to determine if similar effects can be achieved since laboratory rats were utilized in this particular study.

"Intermittent Fasting And Human Metabolic Health"
https://www.ncbi.nlm.nih.gov/pmc/articles/PMC4516560/

Instead of focusing solely on the weight loss benefits that intermittent fasting has to offer, one study, led by the University of California, rather decided to focus on how intermittent fasting would benefit the entire metabolic system of the human body. Instead of doing a separate study, however, the group of researchers who compiled this publication decided to take a look at various existing studies in order to gain an overview of how this diet has affected participants of various studies in the past – and to then make a conclusion as to what health benefits should really be associated with intermittent fasting.

A variety of studies were included in this research project, and their data have been individually reported in the published paper. Below is a quick overview of the data that has been presented here:

- Halberg 2005 study: Eight male patients participated, all of whom were healthy, and none of them were obese. Alternate day fasting techniques were used, with 20-hour fasting windows. The study was conducted over a period of 15 days. Blood glucose levels were significantly reduced by the end of the study. Adiponectin levels rose, and leptin levels were also observed to be much lower than at the start of the study.
- Heilbronn 2005 study: A total of 16 patients participated, half male and half female. All patients were at a healthy weight. The study was conducted over a period of 22 days. There were 36-hour fasting intervals introduced to participants of the study. Insulin levels were significantly reduced at the end of the study.
- Horne 2012 study: There were 30 participants in the study. Twenty of the participants were female, and the rest were male. All participants

were over the age of 18 and healthy. The study was only con-ducted over a period of one single day. Participants were asked to fast for a period of 28 hours, in which they were only advised to consume water. Levels of both LDL cholesterol and HDL cholesterol were increased, while triglyceride levels were observed to be lower by the end of the fasting period. Glucose and insulin levels were also significantly reduced, which provided beneficial effects for individuals with diabetes. There was also a slight decrease in the weight of the individuals who participated in the study.

- Johnson 2007 study: Only 10 participants were included in the study. A total of eight were female, and two were male. All of the patients had asthma and were considered overweight, but not obese. The study was conducted over a period of eight weeks. At the end of the study, body weight was reduced among the participants. There was an increase in HDL cholesterol and a reduction in triglycerides. Two inflammatory markers were also reduced, including BDNF and TNF-a.
- Varady 2009 study: A total of 20 participants were involved in this particular study, with 12 being female and the rest male. The study was conducted over eight weeks, and only obese individuals were involved in the study. Participants experienced a reduction in their body weight, as well as lower triglyceride levels

and LDL cholesterol levels.

CHAPTER 10

FREQUENTLY ASKED QUESTIONS ABOUT INTERMITTENT FASTING

Can I drink coffee while I am fasting?

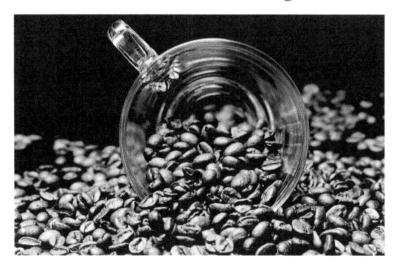

Coffee is a beverage that millions of people enjoy each and every day. This is why many people are concerned that they might have to give up their cup of coffee that they enjoy so much each morning if they are going to start following an intermittent fasting plan – the majority of these plans will tell you to sustain from eating until later in the afternoon and to skip on breakfast for a boost in benefits.

Fortunately, there is no need to worry if you are planning to implement intermittent fasting into your diet – and would still like to have a cup or two of coffee in the morning. There is, however, one particular factor that you do need to note here. If you want to have a cup of coffee after waking up and your intermittent fasting plan demands that you continue with your fasting window in the morning, then it means no sugar and no milk for you. While some people have noted that it is okay to add one splash of milk to your coffee while fasting, this is usually not recommended if you are serious about losing weight while you are following an intermittent fasting plan.

Coffee can actually be a great addition to your diet plan and be a good boost for getting through that last period of fasting. When you opt for a cup of coffee in the morning, you will get an energy boost – and since the caffeine in coffee may provide you with benefits for as long as six hours, you can easily glide on these effects until the time comes to break your fasting period.

Coffee has also been shown to speed up metabolism, which is great for anyone looking to lose weight. You'll end up burning even more fat.

Additionally, coffee will help to keep your mind sharp during the morning and avoid those dreadful times when brain fog hits you because you are running on empty.

There is another benefit that should be noted in terms of having a cup of coffee for breakfast, instead of indulging in a big breakfast. This particular benefit comes in handy for those who are looking to work out while they are still fasting – many people prefer a morning workout, after all. There are some people who follow an intermittent fasting plan that finds they do not have the same level of energy while working out compared to eating a good breakfast before they go out and hit the gym. When you drink some coffee, you'll get a boost in both physical performances, and cognitive function – both of these are crucial for a good workout in the gym.

Should I break my fast with a big or small meal?

Another popular question that people tend to ask when it comes to intermittent fasting is how exactly they should break their fast. The opinions in regards to breaking a fasting window while following an intermit-tent fasting program is mixed. Some suggest that you break the fast with a big meal that is packed with calories to load your body with protein and other essential nutrients, while others suggest that you start out simple and small, and then gradually work up to that big meal.

There really isn't a single perfect answer to this question, but it should be taken into account that when breaking a fast, the body is still in a fat burning mode. When you hit your body with too many calories at once, you can switch off this mode and experience less of the benefits that you are expecting from your intermittent fasting plan.

Thus, it is generally not considered a good idea to break your fast with a meal that is considered loaded in calories. I personally find that it is much more convenient to start things out slowly. Perhaps break that fasting period with a green salad, or perhaps some Greek yogurt. There are many options that can help to satisfy the hunger you have built up during the fast, offer you a series of healthy and essential nutrients, but without causing your metabolism to shut down.

After the fast has been broken and you have had your first meal, plan for a second and a third meal as well. Be sure that these meals will also be nutritious and healthy. I enjoy a big meal that makes up most of the calories I should consume daily by the end of the day. Some might prefer this "big meal" to happen in between their first and third meal – this way, they can start their eating cycle and end the cycle with something small. This would also help to reduce the number of calories you should consume just before you go to bed.

If you are not sure which one you prefer, be sure to consider the various meal plan examples that I have shared with you in this book. You'll find a couple of different meal plans spread out throughout this book – they are all great for those who are starting out without knowing which type of meal plan they would like to implement with their intermittent fasting program.

A good idea would also be to experiment with different options. Try to make the second meal of the eating period your big meal of the day. See how your body reacts. You might also try the first and the final meal of the day – make these your big meals. Really observe how you feel with each of these options. You'll eventually start to notice that your body re-acts better to one of these particular options – or perhaps spreading out your calories equally. When you find the right option, continue with it.

How do I cope with my hunger during the fasting window?

When you are starting out with intermittent fasting for the first time and you are used to eating three or more meals a day, along with some snacking in-between, then there really is no doubt that for the initial period of intermittent fasting, you will experience hunger and some cravings. This is something that most people struggle with – and it is an issue that often causes people to give up on intermittent fasting and either return to their usual way of eating or turn to another type of diet to help them possibly lose the excess weight that is causing them concern.

The key to success in terms of coping with hunger when starting with an intermittent fasting program really is patience. You will need to have patience when it comes to feeling the effects of this diet come into play. It will take some time, but when you push through these hunger strikes, then you will start to notice the cravings become fewer and fewer as the days go by. Instead of experiencing cravings for candy and other un-healthy foods, you will start to experience hunger – this is a good thing, so do not think of the hunger as a bad thing that is striking you at the most unpleasant times.

Since you are not craving unhealthy foods, you will be less likely to start searching for donuts and candy bars to snack on. You'll also find that it is easier to push through until you reach the time where you can have your first meal.

If you do feel that you are unable to cope anymore and those last few hours simply seem too far away, then have sparkling water. This will help to make your stomach feel full for a little while – in turn, and you will find that it becomes much easier to last for an hour or two more in order to reach the time when you can finally break your fast.

How will I train if I am running empty on food?

While coping with hunger is one thing that people struggle with when they are following an intermittent fasting plan, another issue that some also find is that they are not sure how they will continue with their training regimen once they start to follow this type of program. The obvious idea behind intermittent fasting is that you would find yourself running low on food just in the nick of time when you decide to hit the gym – this means you do not have an adequate source of fuel to give you that energy you need to push through the entire session.

In reality, some people actually find that they are able to train more efficiently when their stomach is not full. There are also many who have claimed training during a fasting period is more beneficial – and that it is sometimes even easier.

If you do feel that you are unable to get through that upcoming training session because you feel "empty" and out of energy, then perhaps con-sider opting for a cup of coffee – no milk or sugar, however. The coffee will give you the boost you need to get through the entire session and may even give you some energy afterward to last until the time at which you can break the fast.

Keep in mind that when training on an empty stomach, your body will not have food to turn to in order to generate energy. In turn, this also means that your body will start to turn to the fat storages within your body in order to generate the energy that you need to continue running on that treadmill or to continue pushing those weights. This, in turn, also means fat is burnt faster and much more effectively.

Is it okay to cheat now-and-then?

When it comes to intermittent fasting for weight loss, people are usually inclined to follow a specific meal plan and diet that will give them guidance on what they can eat during the periods that they are allowed to consume calories. In the majority of cases, diets will be somewhat restricted – they will usually include healthy foods that are relatively low in carbohydrates while being high in protein and other essential nutrients.

The healthy meals will surely make you feel great, but there is no shame in wanting to have a "cheat" snack or even a cheat meal now-and-then. The big question now is whether or not it is okay for you to have a cheat day, or even just a cheat snack or treat.

In reality, having a "cheat" day will not do you a lot of harm in terms of your weight loss results – the important part here is to ensure that this does not happen every day. Try to limit yourself to a cheat once a week at most. Perhaps grab a bar of chocolate from your local supermarket or, if you really want to go bigger, get your family to agree to dinner at a local restaurant.

When you do have a cheat day or meal, it is important that you take the calories consumed while 'cheating' into account. This number of calories you will have to make up for the next day – this way, you'll continue to experience the benefits of the diet.

Consider the number of calories you went over your daily limit today – perhaps that bar of chocolate added another 150 calories to your day.

The next day, be sure to reduce your calorie consumption to make up for the excess in calories that you decided to have the previous day.

https://www.ncbi.nlm.nih.gov/pmc/articles/PMC4516560/

CHAPTER 11

CONCLUSION

I hope this book helped you understand the basics of occasional fasting and the benefits that this diet will bring into your life. By practicing occasionally fasting while you are fit, without having to adhere to strict diets that can be harmful to your health, you will succeed in reducing weight and be in the best form of your life.

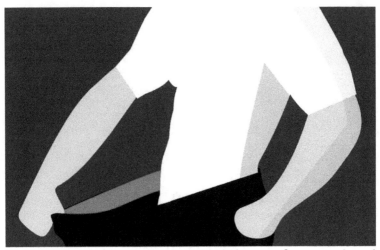

Understanding the principles of occasional fasting, will not only help to reduce your weight, but it will also contribute to the strengthening of your mental health by training your brain to be durable and to resist food in moments that are meant for fasting. This way you will become a stronger person. But the psyche is not the only thing that will be strengthened. Who does not want strong and well-shaped muscles? Well, occasional fasting will help in creating this. You must be wondering how can something that deprives you of food, helps you build muscle when you know that building muscle requires more calorie intake. Well, this is not the case. Basically, intermittent fasting will teach you to appreciate food and to refer to a healthy diet that will become part of your everyday life. With the right combination of fat, carbohydrates, protein, fresh fruits and vegetables, you will able to create meals that the body needs on the days of not fasting.

The next step is to list all the various methods of

intermittent fasting once more, to help you choose the one that will best suit your lifestyle and daily responsibilities, and gradually start to change your life and take care of your health forever. Of course, do not be alarmed if you are suddenly unable to endure the whole fasting period. Allow your body some time to get used to this way of eating, and over time you will be able to lengthen the time for fasting. Combine some simple exercises to increase the burning of fat from your body, or prepare your own exercise plan that will fit your fitness level. But, try not to forget the recommendations given in the book of the combination of the intensity of exercise on the days when you are fasting and the days when you are not fasting.

It is important to plan exercise days well. If you practice high-intensity workouts on the fasting day, you will feel exhausted, and your muscles will be under a lot of stress, which is not good when you are trying to shape and enhance. Also, to get those well established and toned muscles, drink plenty of water (at least eight glasses, but really this is the mini-mum amount we need) and remember to combine protein, carbohydrates, and fat before and after training to help your muscles grow. Take the recommendations for gradual entry into the process of fasting and become one step closer to changing your whole life and becoming happier and satisfied with your visual appearance and health.

www.ingramcontent.com/pod-product-compliance
Lightning Source LLC
LaVergne TN
LVHW012337130725
816069LV00009B/509